RUN LIKE A PRO

(EVEN IF YOU'RE SLOW)

RUN LIKE A PRO

(Even If You're Slow)

Elite Tools and Tips for Runners at Every Level

MATT FITZGERALD AND BEN ROSARIO

BERKLEY

NEW YORK

BERKLEY
An imprint of Penguin Random House LLC
penguinrandomhouse.com

Interior photos by Evan Barnes

Library of Congress Cataloging-in-Publication Data

Names: Fitzgerald, Matt, author. | Rosario, Ben, author.
Title: Run like a pro (even if you're slow): elite tools and tips for
runners at every level / Matt Fitzgerald and Ben Rosario.
Description: First edition. | New York: Berkley, 2022.
Identifiers: LCCN 2021034764 (print) | LCCN 2021034765 (ebook) |
ISBN 9780593201916 (trade paperback) | ISBN 9780593201923 (ebook)
Subjects: LCSH: Sports—Physiological aspects. | Exercise.
Classification: LCC RC1235.F583 2022 (print) | LCC RC1235 (ebook) |
DDC 613.7/1—dc23
LC record available at https://lccn.loc.gov/2021034764
LC ebook record available at https://lccn.loc.gov/2021034765

First Edition: March 2022

Printed in the United States of America

Book design by Pauline Neuwirth

For Jeff Johnson, running legend and so much more.

—Matt Fitzgerald

For my high school coach Jim Linhares, who helped me fall in love with running and remains a role model to this day.

—Ben Rosario

CONTENTS

MATT FITZGERALD AND BEN ROSARIO

RUN LIKE A PRO

(EVEN IF YOU'RE SLOW)

INTRODUCTION

*H*I. MY NAME IS Ben Rosario. But you can call me Coach Ben, as a whole heck of a lot of runners have done for the past twenty years. Let's skip the part where I tell you that I started running in middle school, and then ran cross-country and track in high school, and then ran in college. To be clear, I did all of that, but since this is a book on coaching, it seems more appropriate that I skip ahead to 2003, when, for the first time, I was officially given the Coach Ben moniker.

I was living in Michigan and running (semi)professionally for the Hansons Brooks Original Distance Project, an elite team based in the suburbs of Detroit. For a few hundred bucks, I took a gig as an assistant coach at Van Hoosen Middle School. I worked with the distance runners, naturally (I know nothing about sprinting or field events), and, much to their delight, introduced them to the Swedish word for speed play, *fartlek*.

New vocabulary aside, my approach to coaching those kids was based on a set of principles and methods that I, like most coaches, had borrowed from my own mentors and role models along the way. Things like the importance of form drills, which I learned from my high school cross-country coach Jim Linhares. And the amazing, darn-near-magical powers of long-term aerobic development, which I learned from Coach Dave Barney when I attended the University of Arkansas cross-country camp in 1996. Or the idea of training to race,

1

not training to train, that I learned from my hard-nosed, old-school college coach, Ed Schneider. Not to mention what I learned from my professional coaches, Kevin Hanson and, later, Greg McMillan. So many of the workouts that I have given to athletes at all levels through the years—and a few of which I will share with you in this book—are versions of what I was given by Kevin when I was in Michigan, and by Greg when he coached me in the mid-2000s.

In short, my coaching philosophy is something of a hodgepodge, but while it may lack systematicity, it brings together what I believe to be a wonderful blend of art and science. The science comes from the books, articles, and conferences I have read and attended as well as from hundreds of conversations with my own coaches, and now my coaching colleagues, over the course of nearly thirty years. These things have given me the foundational knowledge necessary to work with endurance athletes.

The art, meanwhile, comes largely from the successes—and the mistakes—I experienced in my own running. Mistakes like hanging on too long to the idea that the more miles you run, the better you'll be. (Not exactly. There's a sweet spot between too little and too much, as I learned from Greg McMillan.) Successes like realizing, late in my career, that I actually had speed—I just hadn't been doing the right things, such as plyometric exercises, to access it. (When I did, I ran a 4:03 mile at the age of twenty-nine, a full seventeen seconds faster than I'd run in college.)

I'm happy to say that my successes have outnumbered my mistakes with the runners I've coached. That's because the methods I've collected over the years simply work, not just for some but for all runners. They worked for those middle schoolers in Michigan. They worked in the two years I spent as an assistant at my old high school, where we finished second and first in back-to-back years at the state cross-country meet. They worked for the beginning runners of all ages and abilities I coached through a running retail store I opened in St. Louis in 2006. They worked for the sub-elite athletes I coached to top-twelve finishes at the Boston and Chicago marathons and to the semifinal round of the women's 800 meters at the 2012 Olympic trials. And, though the stakes are much higher, they have worked for the last eight years in Flagstaff, Arizona, where I've been Coach Ben to a team of professional athletes.

That team, HOKA ONE ONE Northern Arizona Elite (NAZ Elite), has become one of the preeminent training groups in the entire world. We have produced eleven national titles, eight World Marathon Major top-ten finishes, eight world championships appearances, five international medals, and, most recently, our own Aliphine Tuliamuk won the 2020 US Olympic Trials Marathon and competed in the Olympic Games. I am duly proud of all of these accomplishments, but I am equally proud that our team has the privilege of sharing our journey with running fans all over the globe.

In the hope of motivating and inspiring others, we share everything openly—our training, our highs and lows, our victories and our defeats. In 2016, when Matt Fitzgerald, a world-famous author with a reputation for thinking outside the box, invited me to sit down for a cup of coffee before the California International Marathon, it was that openness that he hoped would spur me to say yes to one of his crazy ideas. His pitch was this: At age forty-six, he wanted to move to Flagstaff the following July and spend the next three months training like a pro as he prepared for the 2017 Bank of America Chicago Marathon. I said, "Sure, let's do it."

When Matt came out to Flag, he was quickly introduced to those principles I previously alluded to. He had to do a fartlek, of course, just like the kids at Van Hoosen Middle. And he had to do mile repeats, and monster long runs, and all the workouts that have become staples of our training at NAZ Elite. But there is a whole lot more to it than that. And I think Matt knew there would be. After all, he's been preaching the importance of learning from the pros in his books for almost twenty years. But now he was living it.

Like the pros, Matt woke up early to activate his muscles before each and every run. Like the pros, he had post-run smoothies at the ready after hard workouts. Like the pros, he submitted to strength and conditioning sessions, massages (the not-fun kind), and driving two hours to see one of the most highly regarded physiotherapists in the country. For three months, he was a pro (minus the paycheck).

And, of course, he had a professional coach. I took working with

3

Matt very seriously. I wanted him to feel like a part of the team, and I believed the best way to do that was to make him a part of the team. He was treated like everyone else. We sat down at the beginning of the training segment and talked about how I approach things. I didn't pull any punches then, and I remained honest with him throughout the entirety of his time in Flagstaff. It's my belief that, as a coach, if you are always honest with your athletes, then you are at a huge advantage come race week, because then, when you give them a plan, they will know it's not just talk. They'll know you believe, deeply, in what you are telling them they can do. In turn, they will believe in themselves, sometimes in a way they never thought possible.

Matt's a pretty confident guy, so I can't say he never thought this was possible, but on his race day, in Chicago, at forty-six years of age, he ran the marathon in two hours, thirty-nine minutes, and thirty seconds, smashing his personal best, set nearly a decade earlier. And he proved his hypothesis that emulating the pros can, in fact, make you better. I would simply add that "you" is very much the general you. I realize that Matt's 2:39:30, from a percentage standpoint, is considered way above average. But here's the thing: I've seen similar breakthroughs from runners trying to break three hours in the marathon, and runners trying to break four hours, and so on. Pushing the envelope, trying new things, going to failure, and other similar concepts are not reserved for the elite. They are relative, and they work across the board.

In the years since his crazy experiment, Matt and I have remained friends and we've remained steadfast in our shared belief that any runner on this planet, regardless of talent, or age, or experience, can become better by borrowing a few things from those who run for a living. Not the exact paces or the exact volumes that those athletes run (as much as we might wish we could borrow these), but rather the principles by which they train and live—the principles that have served me well for the last twenty years and that Matt and I now wish to share with you in this book.

So, what do you say: Do you want to run like a pro? Good. Let's do this!

FOLLOW THE
LEADERS

RUNNING IS A UNIQUELY democratic sport. When you line up at the start of, say, the New York City Marathon as a middle-of-the-pack runner, you are standing on the same bridge (the Verrazzano-Narrows) as the professionals, feeling the same nervous tension they feel and hoping to reach the same finish line in Central Park. Such inclusiveness may also be found at events like the USATF Cross Country Championships, where elite and recreational runners alike have the opportunity to test their fitness on the host course. Even made-for-TV competitions such as the Millrose Games feature races for pros, high school athletes, and club runners of all ages. In running, we're all in it together in ways that professional and amateur athletes in other sports are not.

Away from the racecourse, however, the sport of running is oddly divided. In their training methods, eating habits, recovery methods, and other practices, elite and nonelite runners could scarcely be less alike. The pros do most of their running at low intensity, whereas nonelite runners do most of theirs at moderate intensity. The pros perform functional strength workouts designed especially to meet the specific needs of runners, whereas nonelite runners are more likely to eschew strength training altogether or do it in forms like CrossFit or yoga that were not developed with runners in mind. The pros typically maintain a balanced, well-rounded, inclusive, and shtick-free diet based on natural foods of all kinds, whereas nonelite runners more often go for elimination-type diets (like keto, plant-based, or Paleo) that are all about exclusion.

You get the idea. It almost seems as if nonelite runners are deliberately doing the opposite of everything the elites do, though the reality is that, for reasons Coach Ben and I will get into later, most aren't even aware of how the pros balance their intensities, strength train, eat, and so forth. As that rare runner who, in a sense, has a foot in both worlds, elite and nonelite, I am keenly aware of this rift. An amateur runner myself, I coach fellow amateurs, but I also interact with the pros through my writing and can use what I learn from them to help my runners and myself improve.

It's a role I was practically born to fulfill. When I was eleven years old, I became both a runner and a fan of professional running in a single moment. That moment occurred during the 1983 Boston Marathon, when I watched my father complete his first 26.2-miler and saw Joan Benoit record a world-best marathon time for women. My dad's achievement inspired me to follow in his footsteps and run, while Joan's admittedly much greater feat moved me to become an active follower of professional running, beginning with local heroes Lynn Jennings, a three-time world champion in cross country, and Cathy Schiro, a national high school cross country champion and Olympian, both of whom lived minutes away from my family's home in New Hampshire's seacoast region.

It so happened that the coach of the girls' cross country team at the high school I attended was Jeff Johnson, who held the distinction of having been Nike's first employee and who'd formerly rubbed elbows with the likes of Steve Prefontaine and the legendary University of Oregon coach Bill Bowerman. As a member of the boys' team, I was never directly coached by Jeff, but he did mentor me to some degree, instilling in me a better understanding of state-of-the-art training principles than most runners my age possessed.

If Jeff Johnson wasn't your typical high school cross country coach, neither was Tom Donnelly your typical Division III running coach. An All-American performer at Villanova University in the 1960s, Tom went on to become the men's cross country and track coach at tiny Haverford College in Pennsylvania. There, he developed a reputation for turning B-level high school runners like me into collegiate All-Americans while as a side gig also coaching elite runners including Ireland's Marcus O'Sullivan, a three-time world champion at 1500 meters. Unfortunately, I didn't actually run at Haverford, having temporarily burned out on the sport, so Tom's influence on me, like Jeff's, was mostly indirect.

After graduating in 1993, I took my English degree to the San Francisco Bay Area, where I found a job writing for a newly launched endurance sports magazine. Being immersed in this environment drew me back into running and at the same time afforded me a chance to learn directly from world-class endurance athletes and elite-level coaches. Tour de France cyclist Bob Roll, world champion runner Regina Jacobs (later busted for doping, alas), mountain biker Marla Streb, and triathlon coach Phil Maffetone are just a few of the many luminaries I interviewed and wrote about during this period, and I eagerly applied much of the knowledge I acquired to my own training, racing, and overall lifestyle.

By 2001, I felt confident enough in my experience and expertise to start coaching runners and triathletes. Only then did I discover that what seemed obvious to me—that any athlete seeking to get better should take their cues from the champions—wasn't obvious to everyone. Having been taught early on that athletes at all levels should emulate the pros, I hadn't realized that most athletes are not so fortunate, hence know little about the methods they use to prepare for races, much less actually practice these methods. For example, whereas professional runners do lengthy, multimodal warm-ups that include activation exercises, jogging, drills, and strides (short, relaxed sprints) prior to their workouts and races, nonelite runners, by and large, warm up with a bit of jogging and nothing more.

In observing such discrepancies, the sociologist in me (I minored in the subject at Haverford) couldn't help but wonder why amateur runners do just about everything differently from professional runners. The conclusion I've arrived at is that, rather than one big reason, there are many small ones. All of them are surmountable, thankfully, and the first step toward doing so and beginning to run like a pro is understanding these reasons. Let's take that step together now.

REASON #1:
MOST RECREATIONAL RUNNERS
ARE LATE STARTERS

In 1983, when my father completed his first Boston Marathon, running was a very different sport than it is today—a lot smaller and a lot more competitive. Back then there were only a few dozen marathons to choose from in the United States, and although Boston was alone in maintaining strict qualifying standards, self-selection ensured that serious racers were the dominant type at all of them. Indeed, to this day the 1983 Boston Marathon remains the fastest marathon ever staged on American soil, with 316 runners finishing the race in less than two hours and thirty minutes.

Among those runners was Ben Beach, who finished 236th with a time of 2:27:43. Ben was typical of the runners of his day. A Maryland native, he started running competitively in high school in the late 1960s, when the first major "running boom" was just getting started. Had he been born a few years earlier, Ben probably would have done what most youth runners did after receiving their diploma, which was to quit the sport. Instead, when Ben moved north to Boston to study medicine at Harvard, he got caught up in the thriving local running culture and chose to continue training and competing, racing his first Boston Marathon as a college freshman in 1968 (and every Boston Marathon since then).

If the first running boom served mainly to turn former high school and college runners into adult road racers, the second running boom, which began in the mid 1990s, cast a much wider net, bringing men and women from all sport and fitness backgrounds—and with no background whatsoever—into the fold. Oprah Winfrey's successful completion of the 1994 Marine Corps Marathon was a watershed moment, opening the door to competitive running to all-comers.

This welcome explosion in popularity did not come without a downside, however. Folks who discover running as adults are vulnerable to bad influences in a way that younger starters often are not. It's worth noting that the man who coached Oprah to her first (and last) marathon finish, Bob Greene, was a personal trainer who specialized in conditioning for downhill skiing and had no expertise in distance running. Oprah got lucky in choosing a technically unqualified coach who nevertheless did a good job in preparing her for Marine Corps, but all too many adult beginners, not knowing any better, seek guidance from questionable sources that steer them in the wrong direction.

The nub of the problem is running's deceptive simplicity, which leads many people to the mistaken belief that anyone who knows a thing or two about fitness can coach running effectively. If you doubt me, try the following test: Walk into your local CrossFit box and ask the head instructor if he or she can help you train for a marathon. The answer will very likely be yes, and if you follow through on the offer (please don't), you'll end up on a program that's heavy on burpees and light on long runs, which will set you up for an ugly encounter with "the wall" on race day.

Those who get an early start in running are far less likely to fall victim to poor guidance. The better middle and high school track programs are, more often than not, coached by men and women who understand that burpees only get you so far as a distance runner. I myself was all of fifteen years old when Jeff Johnson turned me on to Arthur Lydiard, the legendary New Zealand coach who revolutionized the training of distance runners in the 1950s and whose principles still form the foundation of elite training today. At the college level, coaching standards are even higher, such that it's almost impossible to run competitively through college and graduate not knowing enough to coach yourself, if you so choose.

Again, for adult starters, it's much different. Best practices, like the 80/20 rule of intensity balance (which we'll discuss at length in chapter 4), are not intuitive, and therefore they must be learned by each individual beginner, regardless of age. It took many generations for elite runners themselves to discover such methods through collective trial and error. A good example is tapering, or training lighter before races. As commonsensical as it may seem, this method wasn't widely practiced until the great Czech runner Emil Zátopek won the 1950 European Championships 5000 meters and 10,000 meters after being hospitalized for food poisoning, hence forced to abandon his nor-

9

mal routine of training hard right up until the eve of racing, as was the norm back then.

When I started running as a preteen, I made up my own training program. It entailed running six miles every other day and trying to beat my previous time every time. I lasted about a week and a half before I hit a dead end and had to rethink my approach. Sure, you can blame my fraught start on youthful naivete, but in truth, new runners of any age do pretty much everything wrong in training if they follow the wrong counsel (including their own).

The solution? We'll talk solutions at the end of the chapter. First, though, we need to continue looking at the reasons amateur runners don't run like the pros.

REASON #2:
RUNNING FITNESS IS INVISIBLE

The next time you find yourself at a newsstand, pick up and skim through a bodybuilding magazine. What you'll notice is that most of the training and nutrition articles have a well-known professional bodybuilder as the focal point. For example, you might see a feature on the reigning Mr. Olympia's biceps workout or a write-up about a past Arnold Classic winner's weight-cutting plan. It doesn't matter which particular issue of which magazine you select—they're all the same.

The point I'm making is that in some other sports, such as bodybuilding, recreational participants do consciously emulate the methods used by the professionals, which I think has to do with a natural human bias toward visual proof—the seeing-is-believing factor. The top professional bodybuilders all have gigantic muscles. What more proof does anybody need that their training methods and dietary practices (and, yes, the steroids that many use) are effective?

Not so with running. When a pro runner goes from out-of-shape by his standards (perhaps due to illness) to peak shape by implementing elite best practices, he probably doesn't look much different at the end of the process than at the beginning. Physiological testing would likely show significant improvements in factors such as VO_2max (a measure of the maximum rate at which an athlete is able to consume oxygen during exercise, also known as aerobic capacity—the higher the better) and running economy (the rate at which a runner consumes oxygen at a given speed—the lower the better). Alas, this type of proof doesn't pack the same punch as Charles Atlas–style before and after pictures. The effectiveness of elite methods and practices just isn't that obvious to the average nonelite runner.

REASON #3:
PEER GROUP CONFORMITY /
THE IS-IT-WORTH-IT? PRINCIPLE

In 2017, the *Open Access Journal of Sports Medicine* published a study by researchers from the Cambridge Centre for Sport and Exercise Science comparing training patterns in slower and faster marathon runners. Ninety-seven recreational marathoners completed questionnaires asking for detailed information about their training habits and running history. In addition, all ninety-seven runners underwent physiological testing. To the surprise of no one, the researchers found that faster runners trained a lot more than slower ones. The following table summarizes their findings.

MARATHON TIME	2.5-3 HOURS	3-3.5 HOURS	3.5-4 HOURS	4-4.5 HOURS	4.5-5 HOURS
Average Runs per Week	5.7	5.0	4.1	4.9	4.4
Average Miles per Week	56.9	50.5	38.7	34.8	27.2

There are two ways to interpret this data. On the one hand, it could indicate that training more produces faster marathon times. On the other hand, the same data might suggest that naturally faster marathoners simply choose to train more. As ho-hum as the study's findings themselves may be, they leave open the question of which comes first: more training or faster marathons? My personal belief is that *both* interpretations are true to a certain degree.

Here's something that might surprise you: there is virtually zero scientific research showing that training more results in better run-

11

ning performance. Now, I'm not suggesting that training more doesn't result in better performance. However, executing a study that properly addresses this question is next to impossible. It would require the recruitment of previously untrained individuals into one of two training programs with different amounts of running. Sounds easy enough, right? But here's the rub: beginning runners with low levels of fitness can't tolerate large volumes of running right off the bat, so the two programs would have to start in the same place and slowly diverge in volume over many months, and there isn't an exercise-science department in the world with a budget big enough to incentivize currently unfit individuals to make a long-term commitment to a running program that culminates in huge amounts of running. To my knowledge, such an experiment has never been attempted, and therefore we must rely on real-world evidence to assess the effect of running volume on performance.

Fortunately, plenty of studies of this type do exist. The largest and best of these to date was conducted by Thorsten Emig of Paris-Saclay University and Jussi Peltonen of the Polar Corporation and included training and racing data collected from devices worn by more than fourteen thousand runners for a combined 1.6 million exercise sessions. In a paper published in the journal *Nature* in 2020, Emig and Peltonen reported that their data showed not only a clear correlation between running volume and performance across the subject population but also a strong association between running volume and performance within individual runners.

This last finding is particularly important. A skeptic can always look at data showing a relationship between running volume and performance at a group level and argue that it's just as likely to indicate that faster runners choose to train more as to indicate that running more makes runners faster. But even the stubbornest devil's advocate must concede that when vast numbers of runners are observed to get faster *individually* as they run more, a clear causal connection must exist. Again, though, it's possible that both things are true—that running more makes runners faster and that faster runners run more—and I believe this is indeed the case.

We humans have a well-known tendency to gravitate toward and invest in pursuits for which we show a natural aptitude. Back in high school, my teammates and I used to joke, "Why couldn't we have been good at something fun?" In truth, we were only half joking. Speaking for myself, as much as I loved running, I probably would have stuck with soccer—the glamour sport where I grew up—if I hadn't sucked at every aspect of the game besides running. But in this respect, I was perfectly normal. A number of studies have shown that initial fitness level and perceived exercise self-efficacy are among the strongest predictors of adherence to a new exercise program. In other words, people who already have a bit of a knack for exercise or who at least *feel* they have a knack for it are more likely to stick with the activity.

Extending this principle, we should only expect that, among those who have made the choice to run, those who display a real gift for it will put more time into it than will those of lesser ability. Whether consciously or unconsciously, each runner decides it is either worth it or not worth it to run more than they currently do, and there's every reason to believe that perceived ability is a factor in these calculations.

Reinforcing this self-selection mechanism is the mighty force of peer group conformity. For obvious reasons, runners tend to train with runners of similar ability. There are occasional exceptions, but for the most part, 4:30:00 marathoners don't train with 2:30:00 marathoners. Runners at each general level of ability therefore tend to cluster in peer groups, and in peer groups of all kinds, individual members tend to adopt the habits of those around them. Why do so many CrossFit devotees adhere to a ketogenic diet? Because so many CrossFit devotees adhere to a ketogenic diet! Similarly, individual elite runners train the way they do partly because other elite runners train the same way, and individual nonelite runners train the way they do because other runners of similar ability train that way.

13

REASON #4:
MANY RUNNERS OVERESTIMATE HOW DIFFERENT
ELITE RUNNERS ARE FROM THE REST OF US

Whenever I make the case at running camps and clinics that nonelite runners should train, eat, and think like the pros, there's always someone in the audience who raises a hand and asks some version of the following question: "I run a twenty-five-minute 5K. How can the methods that work for the pros possibly also work for me?"

This question is based on the idea that elite runners are vastly different from the rest of us—a separate species, almost. The truth is that elite runners aren't nearly as different from the rest of us as you might assume. There are really two different kinds of running talent. One is what I like to call walking-around fitness. If you took one hundred third graders who had never done any formal run training and had them all run a timed mile, a few of them would complete the distance faster than the rest. These kids have a high level of walking-around fitness, or innate distance-running ability. The other type of running talent is trainability, which is the capacity to gain fitness in response to training. Returning to the previous example, if you had these same one hundred third graders train for nine weeks and then repeat the timed mile, the results would be somewhat different, with some of the slower runners improving a lot and some of the faster runners improving little.

Research has shown that walking-around fitness is largely rooted in a small number of genes that support aerobic capacity (VO_2max). Trainability comes from a different and more varied set of genes. Obviously, professional runners are blessed with both—they are pretty fast even without training, and they improve significantly with training. But to benefit from training like a pro, you don't need a lot of walking-around fitness. You just need to have some measure of the trainability they have. And guess what: trainability genes are far more widespread in the human population than genes for walking-around fitness. In a 2017 study, Claude Bouchard of the Pennington Biomedical Research Center's Human Genomics Laboratory created a system for scoring trainability based on how many of the relevant genes an

14

individual had. While there was a high degree of interindividual variation, a significantly greater number of subjects (fifty-two) had the highest possible score than had the lowest (thirty-six). In other words, a lot of us nonelite runners are just as trainable as the pros.

But let's suppose you happen to be on the lower end of the spectrum for both kinds of talent. What then? Even in this scenario, emulating the pros represents your best chance of becoming the fastest runner you can be. No matter what genetic predisposition you might have, your training should prepare your body for the specific demands of whichever race you're aiming toward, and the demands are the same for every participant. Studies have shown that some people benefit far more from high-intensity training than they do from low-intensity training. Does this mean that, if you're one of these runners, and you're targeting a marathon, you should train for it by doing a lot of short, high-intensity runs and little to no prolonged running at low intensity? Absolutely not! To do so would be only slightly less absurd than training for a marathon exclusively by lifting weights just because tests show your body responds to strength training better than to cardiovascular exercise in general. A marathon is a prolonged run at low to moderate intensity. Regardless of DNA, you will not be adequately prepared for this challenge unless your training includes a large number of longer runs at these intensities.

This is not to say that individualization in training isn't important. As Coach Ben will explain in a later coach's tip, he trains each member of Northern Arizona Elite a little differently based on their individual strengths, weaknesses, running history, and patterns of response to various stimuli. But this happens at a granular level. At every other level, these runners train the same, because they're all human and they're all training for the same types of events.

REASON #5:
A LOT OF RUNNERS MISUNDERSTAND WHAT IT MEANS TO TRAIN (AND LIVE) LIKE A PRO

The next time a fellow runner expresses frustration about her lack of improvement, you might suggest, "Hey, I think you should train like a pro." I'm willing to bet her reply will be something along the lines of, "Are you joking? If I tried to run one-hundred-plus miles in one week I would end up in the hospital!" But training like a pro doesn't necessarily mean running one-hundred-plus miles per week. Rather, it means adhering to *the general principles* behind practices such as one-hundred-plus-mile training weeks.

For example, the principle underlying the practice of running one-hundred-plus miles per week is to run a lot relative to one's personal limits. Elite runners, by virtue of their trainability, youth, low body weight, good biomechanics, and experience, have a high personal limit for running volume, and that's why they run one-hundred-plus miles per week. Most other runners have a lower limit, but they still can and should adhere to the principle of running a lot relative to their limit.

The same is true of non-training aspects of the professional-runner lifestyle, such as sleeping upward of ten hours a day (including afternoon naps). The underlying principle to emulate here is that of consistently getting all the sleep you need. Pro runners happen to need upward of ten hours of sleep a day, and chances are you don't. But it's also likely that you don't consistently get all the sleep you need, so you still stand to benefit from adhering to professional principles.

In the same vein, eating like a pro does not necessarily mean eating five thousand calories a day. What it does mean is emulating the core eating habits that are practiced with surprising consistency by elite runners all over the world, a topic we'll address thoroughly in chapter 8.

I could offer additional examples, but I think I've made my point: living like a professional runner is a lot more doable than a lot of nonelite runners think.

REASON #6:
MOST RUNNERS ARE NOT RUNNING FANS

At the beginning of this chapter, I mentioned that I became a runner and a fan of professional running almost simultaneously at age eleven. This is not the norm, of course. A majority of runners who come to the sport as adults take a casual interest at best in elite-level competition. They might follow a few pros on Instagram or read the occasional book authored by an Olympic hero, but they do not (as I do) subscribe to FloTrack so they can watch events like the NCAA cross country championships live or set an alarm for 2:00 a.m. so they can witness a world-record attempt in the half marathon somewhere in Europe.

In times past, such fanaticism wasn't so unusual. The pursuit of the first sub-four-minute mile in the 1940s and '50s, for example, captivated the entire world, generating front-page headlines everywhere from New York to Sydney. But when Daniel Komen of Kenya ran *back-to-back* sub-four-minute miles in 1997, only nerds like me took notice. Unlike football or basketball, the sport of running today is participatory rather than fan-based. Which is not a bad thing, but it is one more reason why nonelite runners tend not to emulate the methods the pros employ in pursuit of better performance. Simply put, the average nonelite runner doesn't pay much attention to the pros, and therefore the average nonelite runner doesn't know much about what the pros do.

I'll give you an example. Relatively few professional runners monitor their heart rate regularly in training. When I mention this to the runners I coach, they are often surprised. I'm not suggesting that you immediately chuck your heart rate monitor (supposing you have one) or put it up for sale on eBay. I'm just underscoring the point that you can't very well do what the pros do if you don't even know what the pros do. And few nonelite runners know much about what the pros do (other than that they run one-hundred-plus miles per week!).

CLOSING THE GAP

As we've seen, there are a lot of reasons nonelite runners tend not to do what professional runners do in pursuit of improvement, yet none of these six reasons should present an insurmountable barrier stopping runners like you from following the leaders, so to speak. Just because you may have started running as an adult and thereby missed the indoctrination in best practices that many high school and college runners receive does not mean you can't learn and adopt these practices now. Likewise, just because—due to the invisibility of running fitness—you might not have fully appreciated how pro runners maximize their fitness does not mean you can't now adopt these techniques to boost your running performance more effectively than any alternatives might. Nor should your perceived talent level stop you from training like the pros just because the runners around you don't train like the pros.

The moment you realize that you're not as different from the elites as you thought, the assumption that their way of training is impossible for you loses any power it has to prevent you from adopting a pro-style training approach. Up to this point, you may have had the wrong idea about what it really means to do what the pros do, assuming it looks like running one hundred miles per week and sleeping ten hours a day when in actuality it's about adhering to the *principles* that inform such practices. If you aren't the biggest fan of elite-level running, and consequently don't know a lot about their methods, you've come to the right place. We're going to show you these methods, which you can adopt if you're serious about improving. All you have to do is buy into the notion that what works for the best athletes in the world can work for you too.

I'm confident that you wouldn't even be reading these words if you weren't serious about improving, and I'm equally confident that, if you aren't already persuaded that emulating the pros is your surest path toward improvement, you're at least on your way. So, let's now turn our focus to the specifics of what it really means to run like a pro.

Coach's Tip

You Are Not as Different from the Elites as You Think

S till not convinced you can (and should) train like the pros? Let me tell you a story.

In 2012, I coached a pair of runners who, on paper, couldn't have been more different. One was a high school state champion and a multiple All-Big 12 performer at the University of Missouri. The other was a guy who had never run a step in his life when I first met him. Yet both men proudly competed for the same retail racing team, Big River Running Company. And both achieved their marathon dreams by following training plans I created for them with a single set of principles and methods.

Matt Gibbs might never have become a runner if he hadn't won a gift certificate for Big River at a holiday party hosted by a local radio station. When Gibbs (as we liked to call him) walked into the store the following week to use that gift certificate, he was out of shape and overweight at just twenty-three years of age. Nevertheless, we gave him the royal treatment—taking him through a full gait analysis, bringing out a bunch of different shoe options, and allowing him to run outside in each pair, all the while chatting with him about running, our community, and the various ways he could get involved. He walked out of the store with a great pair of shoes, but more important, he left excited to give this running thing a try.

Around the same time Gibbs was taking his first steps as a runner, another local twentysomething, Adam MacDowell, was taking his first steps in a running comeback. I had known Adam since I was a freshman in high school, when he was a sophomore at a rival school and a member of the same club team I ran for in the off-season. Adam was one of the area's best runners throughout his high school career, eventually going undefeated during his senior cross-country season en route to becoming state champion. He was recruited by Division I colleges all over the nation before accepting an athletic scholarship at the University of Missouri, where he led the Tigers to three straight trips to the NCAA cross country championships. Like many collegiate athletes, though, Adam was ready for a break when he graduated. That break took the form of an extended stint as a "ski bum" (his words) in Colorado. Being a ski bum does involve some exertion, but for many, including Adam, it also involves lots of beer, and when he returned to Saint Louis in 2005, his fitness was far from the elite level it had been at when he left.

Adam probably would have started running again regardless, but as it happened, his comeback was initiated by a phone call from yours truly, in which I invited him to become a founding member of the Big River Running Company Racing Team (we needed anyone we could get at the time, but Adam was at the top of my list). He said yes almost before I'd finished making my pitch, and the long climb back toward elite fitness began.

In many ways, Adam and Gibbs were in the same boat. One was starting over, the other starting out, and both soon decided they wanted to see what they could do at the marathon distance. What's more, I was their coach, and I know only one way to coach a runner, whether they're an overweight beginner, a former state champion, or anything in between.

When I sat down to write marathon training schedules for Gibbs and Adam, I asked myself the same question: What workouts does this athlete need over the course of the coming training segment to be ready on race day? And although the specifics differed, the work-outs themselves often looked nearly identical. Adam had never run a marathon before. Sure, he'd had a lot of success at shorter distances

20

on the track and on the grass, but he'd need to get his legs callused for 26.2 miles on the roads. Gibbs had never run a marathon either, of course, and his legs would also need to be callused. Thus, I prescribed long runs every weekend for both of them.

I am a believer in adding some "spice" to the long run, so both Adam and Gibbs were required to do "fast finish" long runs, in which the last three miles were much faster than the preceding twelve to fifteen miles. Adam was running those fast miles close to five minutes flat, Gibbs about 30 percent slower, but having seen them at the end of those runs, I can assure you their effort level was very similar.

Perhaps you're thinking that, whereas their long runs may have been alike, surely their "speed work" was vastly different. Nope. Both, for example, hit the track to run 10 x 800 meters fast with a 400-meter jog recovery. The only difference was that "fast" for Adam was 2:20 per 800, compared to 3:20 per 800 for Gibbs.

It is true that Adam ran a lot more than Gibbs overall. Naturally efficient, Adam could handle ninety miles per week in marathon training. Gibbs, not as efficient, and thus at a higher risk for injury, was kept a little lower. But the underlying principle was the same: find the sweet spot where the athlete can run as many miles as possible while still being able to complete the hard workouts successfully and while remaining healthy.

After several years of dedicated training, Gibbs bore little resemblance to the couch potato who walked into my store in search of free stuff. Like the pros, he was running a lot relative to his personal limit. Like the pros, he was challenging himself by running with people of equal or greater ability. Like the pros, he had found his optimal racing weight through sensible dietary improvements. Like the pros, when he had a big race coming up, he got locked in mentally and emotionally. And, like the pros, he succeeded. Gibbs's first marathon was well north of four hours, but he has since lowered his personal record (PR) to 3:19 and moved up to ultramarathons.

Adam, too, achieved his marathon dreams. After a couple of years spent getting back into the groove of training, he got the itch to really commit. His first marathon was the 2011 Chevron Houston Marathon, which he completed in 2:22:16. At that time, the Olympic trials standard was 2:19:00—we realized he had a shot. Not many runners qualify for the trials for the first time at age thirty-two, but Adam was getting better and better. In the fall of 2011, at the Bank of America Chicago Marathon, with his coach (that's me!) pacing him through the midpoint, Adam ran 2:18:47. A little over three months later, the 2012 Olympic marathon trials were held in Houston. And there, this former ski bum and full-time teacher, a guy who hadn't run a marathon until he was in his thirties, finished thirty-seventh in a field of more than one hundred of the country's best marathoners with a personal-best time of 2:17:27.

The moral of the story is obvious. When Matt says that the methods the best runners use to succeed are the best methods for every runner chasing success, he's not just blowing hot air. It's really true, and real runners like Matt Gibbs and Adam MacDowell and the many others I've had the privilege of guiding toward success, however they define it, with a single tool kit, are living proof. So take good notes as Matt and I share the details of this tool kit in the chapters ahead!

PLAN LIKE A PRO

*I*F YOU ASK TEN elite running coaches to describe their training philosophies, you're likely to get ten different answers. How do I know? Because folks like me who write about the sport often ask elite running coaches to describe their training philosophies, and the very reason we keep asking is that we keep getting different answers!

Keith and Kevin Hanson, for example, who coached Ben Rosario during his professional running career, place a strong emphasis on running lots and lots of miles. In contrast, James Li, who for many years coached collegiate athletes at the University of Arizona as well as elite runners from Africa and now heads a running club in his native China, puts less emphasis on mileage and more on intensity. Meanwhile, Renato Canova, an Italian coach who has guided a long list of Kenyan runners to international success, advocates a training process that starts at the extremes of intensity and, over time, works toward the middle (specifically race intensity). But Gjert Ingebrigtsen, who coaches a world-beating trio of his own sons in Norway, believes in avoiding the moderate-intensity range, loading the boys' schedules with sessions of long intervals done slightly above anaerobic threshold intensity. And Steve Magness, who, until recently, served as a cross country and track coach at the University of Houston, trains a handful of elite runners scattered in disparate locations and is known for his "leave nothing behind" approach, where all types of training are kept in the mix throughout the training process.

Running journalists aren't the only ones who know that no two elite running coaches share precisely the same approach to training. So do professional runners, which is why they sometimes change coaches in search of better performance. A case in point is Galen Rupp, a two-time Olympic medalist for the United States who was thirty-three years old and had been running competitively since high school when he started working with Flagstaff-based coach Mike Smith. It wasn't until then that Galen completed his first-ever fartlek run. Evidently this classic, bread-and-butter workout wasn't part of his previous coach's playbook!

You might be asking yourself, *How the heck am I supposed to train like the pros if the pros don't have a well-defined way of training?* Don't worry—they do. It's just that the elite way of training allows for some flexibility. No matter who you are, if you want to be the best runner you can be, there are certain things you *must* do in your training and certain other things you must *not* do, and despite superficial differences, you can be sure that elite runners everywhere obey the cardinal dos and don'ts of training. It's sort of like eating healthy. If you want to maximize the health benefits you get from the food you eat, there are certain habits you must adhere to in your diet and certain other habits you must avoid. But two people with different tastes, preferences, lifestyles, and cultural backgrounds can both stick to all the unbreakable rules of healthy eating without ever eating any of the same specific foods.

Science offers strong support for the idea that there is more than one way to train effectively for distance-running events. One good example is a study conducted by researchers at the University of Western Australia and published in the *Journal of Strength and Conditioning Research* in 2018. The subjects were thirty recreational runners who were separated into three groups. One group practiced so-called linear periodization for a period of twelve weeks, doing high-volume, low-intensity training for six weeks and then switching to low-volume, high-intensity training for six weeks. A second group did the reverse, while a third group served as controls, continuing to do their normal training for twelve weeks. All the subjects completed a 5000-meter time trial both before and after the twelve-week intervention. On average, members of the linear periodization group improved their 5K time by 1:16, while members of the reverse linear periodization group saw a bump of 1:52, and the controls, as expected, stayed the same, trimming a mere three seconds off their initial marks.

The small difference in improvement between the linear and reverse linear groups was judged by the researchers to be statistically insignificant, meaning it was likely a matter of chance. Thus, they concluded, "These results do not support linear periodization or reverse linear periodization as a superior method; however, [both types of] periodized training elicited greater improvements in endurance performance than non-periodized training, highlighting the importance of planned training structure." You couldn't ask for a clearer demonstration of the idea that there is more than one way to train effectively as a runner—and yet not all ways are equally effective.

The crucial characteristic that the two periodization plans shared, and the other program lacked, was—as the study's authors pointed out—*planning*. Cosmetic differences aside, the thing that every elite running coach does with every athlete is plan their training in accordance with proven principles of fitness development. To fulfill your potential as a runner, you must either do the same for yourself or find a coach who understands these principles to do the planning for—or, better yet, *with*—you. Regardless of which path you choose—self-coaching or working with a coach—it's important that you know and understand these principles. The training process always yields better results when the athlete fully buys into the process, and all runners, even those with coaches, have to make some decisions for themselves. You'll make better decisions if you have a basic knowledge of how to plan like a pro.

THE FIVE RULES OF PRO-STYLE PLANNING

There are, by my count, five unbreakable rules of training for competitive distance running. These rules represent the broad principles that all elite running coaches apply to the process of preparing their athletes for competition. By no means do they constitute a complete blueprint for training. They merely provide a general framework for the specific methods and practices that fill out the plan. We'll discuss these methods and practices in the coming chapters. For now, let's stay focused on the bigger picture.

RULE #1—Start Where You Are

At any given time, the highest-performing members of Coach Ben's professional running team are those who've been with it the longest. This is no accident. Developing as a runner takes time. You can't do the training that's necessary to fulfill 100 percent of your potential until you've done the training that prepares you to do that training (a phenomenon sometimes referred to as *training to train*). Each successfully completed cycle of training changes your body, preparing it to take on a little more work in the next cycle. Elite Kenyan running coach Patrick Sang likes to say that he puts each new athlete he adds to his team on a ten-year plan. No amount of innate talent can enable a younger or less experienced runner to skip the development process and jump straight from beginner-level training to advanced—you've got to earn it.

Nonelite runners often don't quite grasp the idea that experience rather than ability should determine how they train, and as a result, they make mistakes. Every so often, I am contacted by a runner seeking help in choosing one of the many training plans I sell through 80/20 Endurance, my online coaching business. These queries always include information that the runner assumes will help me recommend the right plan, often mentioning either a goal time for the runner's next race or his personal best (PB) time at that distance.

Goal times and PBs are not a good basis for selecting a training plan, however. To understand why, consider the hypothetical example of a runner who wants to run a marathon in 3:45:00 and comes to me asking which specific marathon plan I would recommend for this particular goal. If I knew this and only this bit of information about the runner, and if I didn't know what I know about running, I might recommend a plan that features six runs per week and builds up to fifty-five miles of weekly running. But what if the runner seeking my help has never run more than four times per week and more than forty total miles in a single week? In that case, the plan I've steered him toward might be overwhelming. On the other hand, what if the runner has consistently run seven times per week and as much as sixty-five miles in a single week without ever feeling overwhelmed? In this case, the plan I've recommended is likely to take him backward rather than forward.

The point of this hypothetical example is that there is no single training plan that fits every runner pursuing a given goal. Okay, fine. So what *is* the appropriate basis for training-plan selection? Simple: training history. The one goal that every athlete shares is improvement, which tends to occur in modest increments and is made possible by modest increases in *training load* (a variable that factors together the volume and the intensity of training). Your next training plan should therefore administer a training load that is slightly greater than the heaviest training load you handled successfully in preparing for a prior race of the same distance you're targeting this time around. For example, if you built up to forty-five miles per week in preparing for your last marathon, consider building up to fifty miles in preparation for the next marathon.

RULE #2—Choose a Direction

The purpose of training is to make you fitter (duh). To do this, your program has to change over time. You can't do the same training week in and week out and expect to keep getting fitter. Your training must instead move in a clear trajectory that serves to reliably nudge your fitness level in the direction of full race readiness.

The common term for the practice of giving the training process directionality is *periodization*. The first periodization model that achieved worldwide influence in elite running was developed by Arthur Lydiard in the 1950s. It represented what became known as a linear periodization model (an example of which we saw at the beginning of the chapter), meaning it tended to segregate the various training types into separate phases. The first of these was a base phase that consisted of increasing amounts of easy running. Next came a strength phase dominated by hill work, then a speed phase marked by high-intensity interval workouts, and finally a racing phase. Lydiard's system is widely credited with sparking a revolution in elite performance standards affecting every race distance from 800 meters to the marathon. But as it spread across the globe, this system began to mutate and evolve, giving rise to an array of different approaches to periodization, including nonlinear models in which the various training types are mixed together throughout the cycle and only the amounts and proportions change.

Today it is clear that there is no single "best" approach to periodization, as the success of elite coaches who favor slightly different approaches illustrates, and as studies like the University of Western Australia study I described earlier affirm. But this does not mean that all approaches are equally effective. A closer inspection of the training philosophies of elite running coaches reveals that, underneath their surface-level differences, all of them share two bedrock qualities that represent the two things the training process must do to achieve the goal of building maximum fitness.

First, the training process must exhibit a general trend toward increased training load. Simply put, you cannot get fitter as a runner without working harder (unless you're already working too hard). To stimulate the physiological adaptations that increase fitness, you need to subject your body to challenges that are somewhat greater than it is accustomed to. If you run five easy miles every day, another easy five-mile run will not increase your fitness. But an easy six-mile run will, as will a fast four-mile run. And when your body becomes accustomed to easy six-mile runs and fast four-mile runs, you'll need to raise the bar again—a practice that scientists refer to as progressive overload and that elite runners everywhere rely on to improve, regardless of which particular flavor of periodization their coach may favor.

Let's look at an example. This table shows two sample weeks from NAZ Elite member Aliphine Tuliamuk's buildup to the 2020 US Olympic Trials Marathon, which she won. The left column presents the work she did twelve weeks out, at the beginning of the cycle; the right column shows the work she did three weeks out, at the peak of the cycle.

TWO SAMPLE WEEKS OF A
PRO RUNNER'S MARATHON TRAINING

	TWELVE WEEKS OUT	THREE WEEKS OUT
Monday	4 miles easy	10 miles easy 4 miles plus drills and strides (i.e., relaxed sprints)
Tuesday	8 miles easy	12 miles with 20 x 300 meters fast 4 miles easy
Wednesday	12 miles with 20 x (1:00 fast/1:00 easy)	10 miles easy
Thursday	8 miles easy	10 miles easy 4 miles easy
Friday	8 miles easy 4 miles easy	8 miles easy 4 miles plus drills and strides
Saturday	20 miles with 8 x 2:00 at half-marathon pace	20 miles with 15 miles at marathon pace
Sunday	8 miles easy	10 miles easy
Total Mileage: Percentage of Total at Moderate/High Intensity:	72 miles ≈ 14	97 miles ≈ 20

Science confirms what pros like Aliphine know from experience: progressive overload works. Researchers have developed a variety of mathematical tools to quantify training loads that have proven to be reliable predictors of performance. Perhaps the best-known tool of this sort is Eric Banister's training impulse (TRIMP), which uses heart rate data to score the fitness level of individual athletes based on their recent training. In one study, Italian researchers placed eight runners on an eight-week progressive training program and measured changes in both their TRIMP scores and their performance in various fitness tests. As expected, they found that as training loads went up, so did performance. In fact, the researchers reported a correlation coefficient of 0.82 between TRIMP values and performance in a 10,000-meter time trial (0.7 is considered strong, 1.0 perfect).

29

The second thing the training process must do, in addition to get harder, is become more specific to the particular demands of the race event a runner is preparing for. This is because there are many different kinds of fitness. Obviously, the type of fitness that, say, a strongman competitor needs is vastly different from the type of fitness a runner needs, but it's also the case—albeit to a lesser degree—that the type of fitness a marathon runner needs is different from the type of fitness a miler needs. Specifically, a marathoner requires greater endurance and a higher fat-burning capacity, whereas a miler requires greater fast-twitch muscle fiber development and a higher anaerobic capacity.

Because fitness is event-specific, elite running coaches tend to prescribe increasingly event-specific work as a training cycle goes along. You can see this also in Aliphine Tuliamuk's training for the 2020 US Olympic Trials Marathon. The hardest run she did three weeks out from race day was a twenty-miler with fifteen miles at marathon pace—you can't get much more marathon-specific than that. For comparison's sake, consider the workout Aliphine's teammate Danielle Shanahan did eleven days before wrapping up her 2019 season with an indoor 5000-meter race at Boston University. It consisted of four sets of 3 x 200 meters at VO_2 max pace with 200-meter jog recoveries, with each set followed by 400 meters at VO_2 max with a 400-meter jog recovery. For Danielle, VO_2 max pace is 4:45 per mile, which is a little faster than 5000-meter-race pace, and she completed a total of 4000 meters of running at that pace in this particular workout. By design, this session was highly specific to the race that awaited her at BU, where she set a new PB of 15:26.

Did Danielle and Aliphine have to complete these exact workouts to perform as well as they did in their respective races? Absolutely not. Again, it's not the details that matter in training. What *does* matter is that your training becomes harder and more race-specific as you move toward an important race.

RULE #3—(Almost) Always
Do Less than You Think You Could

In a 2011 interview for *Runner's World*, Rhode Island–based elite running coach Ray Treacy said something that I liked so much I immediately shared it on Twitter: "When I hear someone say, 'I just had the best workout of my life,' I get scared. It probably means they just ran their race in practice."

These words pretty well sum up the current elite approach to managing training loads. Some nonelite runners might assume that the pros are constantly testing the limits of how much their bodies can handle, and while there was a time when this was relatively common, today it's rare. History has shown us that testing limits in training seldom ends well, and though most pro runners like to work hard, they like success even more, and so, as a rule, they are careful not to work too hard.

In a book about marathon legend Eliud Kipchoge, Tait Hearps and Matt Inglis Fox describe the restraint that Eliud and his teammates demonstrated in training for the 2017 Berlin Marathon, writing, "Eliud seldom seemed to reach a point where he was maximally exerted. I can't recall a grimace on his face during a workout. He and the other athletes worked very hard, however they methodically trained in a way that gradually built fitness, refraining from all-out efforts and retaining reserves of energy for the most critical of exertions, when it mattered most."

Tom "Tinman" Schwartz, who specializes in coaching top-flight high school runners, has said that his training philosophy can be boiled down to one brief sentence: "Keep the ball rolling." Effective training does not require heroic workouts or brutal weeks. Rather, it's about patient, steady forward progress. Sure, there are times when it's okay to suffer a bit, but for the most part, every runner, whether elite or nonelite, should feel pretty good throughout the training process. Indeed, studies have shown that when athletes begin to feel lousy more often than they feel good, reductions in performance and fitness are just around the corner.

Although nonelite runners don't train as hard as the pros in absolute terms, they actually tend to train harder in relative terms, spending less time feeling good and more time feeling lousy. A large percentage of them think they're *supposed* to feel kind of lousy in training. I can't tell you how many times clients of mine have emailed me to say (in so many words), "Coach, I've been following the plan you gave me and feeling really good. I'm worried it's too easy and I should be doing more." Left to their own devices, many runners will keep training harder and harder until they feel kind of lousy most of the time. To them, this indicates that the training is now hard enough, when in fact it indicates that it's *too* hard.

Here's a good way to avoid this mistake: when you sit down to plan out your next training cycle, create a schedule that represents the limit of what your body can handle without breaking down. Then crumple it up, toss it into the recycling bin, and create a plan that's 10 to 20 percent easier.

RULE #4—Don't Race Too Often

Even though professional runners are paid to race, they don't race very often. A good example is Geoffrey Kamworor, a Kenyan runner who formerly held the half-marathon world record. Geoffrey competed just six times in all of 2019, placing third in the World Cross Country Championships in March, winning a road ten-miler in May, claiming a pair of Kenyan championship titles on the track in July and August, setting his half-marathon world record (58:01) in September, and winning the New York City Marathon in November. That's it.

In the past, things were different. Bill Rodgers raced thirty times in 1978. What changed? The answer is quite simple: money. Until 1982, the governing bodies of the sport of running forbade athletes from receiving compensation from sponsors or race organizers. But, many race organizers paid athletes small appearance fees under the table, incentivizing top runners like Bill Rodgers to race often. Now that sponsorships represent the main income source for pro runners, they not only can afford to compete infrequently but also insist on it, because what they're really being paid for is not to race but to race *well*, and frequent racing is detrimental to performance.

The problem with frequent racing is that it disrupts the flow of training. In order to race well, you need to lighten up your training in the days leading up to the event, and in order to recover properly from racing, you need to lighten up your training for a few days after the event. In total, then, a full week of normal training must be sacrificed for each race. Therefore, it's just not possible to cram multiple races into a short span of time and still do the training required to attain peak performance in any single race. Either you find yourself doing little else besides tapering, racing, and recovering, or you try to train normally despite racing often and your races become nothing more than hard workouts done with a number on your chest.

The exact amount of racing that qualifies as "too much" depends on the distance. Shorter races such as 5Ks require less recovery than do longer races such as marathons. With good planning, you can race a 5K every other week or so for perhaps eight weeks before you start to see a decline in fitness and performance. At the marathon distance, you *might* be able to complete two marathons in six weeks at roughly the same level of performance if you're very fit and highly durable, and even then, you'd need to give yourself at least three months to recover and build a fresh base of fitness before you could complete another marathon at the same level.

Over-racing is one of the more common mistakes that nonelite runners make. I often find myself trying to persuade the runners for whom I build custom training plans to pare down the racing schedules they propose in the onboarding questionnaire they fill out for me. It's not always easy. I've heard runners come up with all kinds of excuses for over-racing: "I need to race a lot to know where I am with my fitness." "I always seem to choke when I put too much focus on any single event." "When I try to go for long periods without racing I tend to overtrain." But these excuses are just that: excuses. Like I've said, we nonelite runners aren't so different from the pros. If frequent racing is harmful to their performance, it's harmful to ours as well.

Some runners don't care about performing at their peak level in every race, and I get that. Chasing PBs isn't the only valid reason for

33

pinning a bib to your singlet. Just don't try to have it both ways. Make a conscious choice either to race sparingly and successfully like the pros or to race often with less success if that's your preference during a particular phase of your running journey.

RULE #5—Rest and Take Breaks

Most runners think of training and rest as opposites. The more you train, the less you rest. Professional runners recognize that rest actually enables them—or any runner—to train more. Ask yourself what the hardest run you could do every single day, year-round, without burning yourself out would be. Not very hard, right? Now think about how much harder your hardest runs could be if you surrounded them with much lighter runs and took a day off every so often. In this manner, rest does not come at the expense of more training but rather creates the possibility for more training.

Rest can take two forms. Absolute rest means not exercising. Relative rest means exercising less than normal. Pro runners typically make far heavier use of relative rest than of absolute rest. An exception is former women's marathon world-record holder Paula Radcliffe, who rested every eighth day throughout the latter part of her storied career. The norm among pro runners is to get relative rest in the form of a single, short recovery run once a week and absolute rest in the form of a day off once every three or four weeks or as needed. This works out just fine most of the time, because if a normal training day for a given pro runner consists of two runs totaling at least twelve miles and often including some work at higher intensities, then doing a single, slow, six-mile run every seventh day will probably give them all the rest their body needs to keep going.

Nonelite runners tend to lean too much on absolute rest and not enough on relative rest. Absolute rest is a blunt instrument—on a given day, you either run or you don't. But relative rest allows you to manipulate your training load in subtler (and more effective) ways. The pros typically use *recovery weeks* rather than days off to ensure they get as much rest as they need but no more. Specifically, every third or fourth week, instead of taking their training load up another notch, they reduce it by around 30 percent for the entire week. This extended, fractional reduction in training is much better than the hard stop of absolute rest. Recovery weeks allow a runner to train and rest at the same time, and for this reason they constitute another way of safely reaching a higher peak training load than would be attainable otherwise.

The following figure is taken from a case study involving three elite Canadian marathon runners conducted by Trent Stellingwerff. It graphs variations in training load over the course of a sixteen-week training cycle. As you can see, it shows an undulating pattern of general increase followed by a taper. The dips preceding the final taper represent recovery weeks. You can be sure that the athletes included in the study took few days off throughout the cycle. The dips resulted from relative, not absolute, rest.

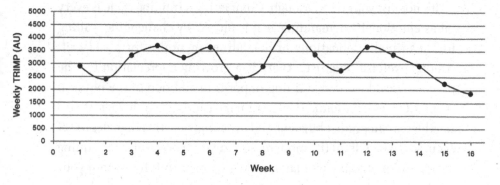

If you're a newer runner, you may *need* to take one or more days off every week to keep your fatigue level from getting out of hand. But newer runners don't stay new forever, and as you build fitness you may find that you can make even more progress if you gradually shift from relying on absolute rest to using relative rest to keep your fatigue level in check.

In addition to building planned rest into their training cycles, pro runners take breaks between cycles. Paula Radcliffe didn't run a step for two weeks after each track season or marathon. Some pros chill out even longer than two weeks, others not as long. Some do no formal exercise whatsoever during breaks, while others enjoy a little light running or alternative activities such as hiking and skiing. But in one way or another, all pro runners take time to regenerate physically and emotionally before starting the next buildup.

When you plan and execute a training cycle properly, you simply *need* a break when it ends. As I mentioned earlier in the chapter, your training load should gradually increase (except in recovery weeks) as the cycle unfolds. In the ideal scenario, this process will culminate in a one- to two-week period of *functional overreaching*, which is a fancy term for training at a level that would burn you out if you tried to sustain it for any length of time but is beneficial in the short run. After that, you taper down and run as hard as you possibly can on race day. By the time you cross the finish line, the major systems of your body (musculoskeletal, cardiovascular, endocrine, immune, and nervous) are far from equilibrium and need a good, solid rest to get back there.

It's not just your body, though. Completing a training cycle is every bit as emotionally demanding as it is physically challenging, calling for sustained applications of discipline, mental effort, and grit. Among exercise scientists, there is a growing appreciation for the psychological load that training imposes in addition to the physical stress. Studies have found that certain measures of psychological load in athletes can predict burnout and even injury with a high degree of accuracy, which is all the more reason to take a break after a training cycle, and preferably one lasting long enough to fully restore your motivation and enthusiasm for running. At the beginning of a break, many pros can't bear the thought of completing another training cycle. But by the end, they can't wait to start getting after it again.

Nonelite runners are far more likely to try to "keep the momentum going," as they often put it, after completing a training cycle. It's understandable. You've worked hard to cultivate a high level of fitness—why give it away? This get-fit-stay-fit mind-set is a carryover from the general fitness realm, where a lot of runners get their start. In a typical scenario, somebody decides they need to lose a few pounds, signs up for a gym membership, and starts working out. At first, they can't handle a lot of exercise so they don't do a lot. But as they get fitter, they do more and more, until they reach a point where they're either seeing the results they want or they've run out of motivation to do more, so they lock into a routine and try to sustain it.

This approach works well for goals like losing weight and improving overall health. But runners need to train in a more progressive manner, building toward performance peaks that create the need for a period of rest. At these times—counterintuitive though it may be—the best move a runner can make to ensure they're even fitter for their next big race is to give away some of that hard-earned fitness. The pros do it and so should you.

How often are breaks needed? It depends. Twenty-four weeks is about the maximum length of time any runner can train in a progressive manner without burning out. If you start a training cycle relatively unfit and you're training for a longer event such as a marathon, you may need a full twenty-four weeks to get race ready and earn a break. But a training cycle can and often should be a lot shorter—ten to twelve weeks—if you start it with good fitness and/or you're training for shorter events.

FROM FRAMEWORK TO BLUEPRINT

Let's quickly summarize what we've learned about the rules that professional runners follow in planning their training.

First, they start where they are in terms of their fitness and experience. The first week of each new training cycle is only slightly more challenging in volume and intensity than the training that preceded it. Likewise, the hardest week of the training cycle is no more than moderately harder than the hardest week of the last one, and the paces and times the pros target throughout the cycle reflect their current fitness level, not their goals.

Second, each training cycle has a clear direction, and in particular, it exhibits a clear trend toward increased training loads and a progression from general to specific, with key workouts becoming more and more particular to the next big race.

But third, while the pros' training gets progressively harder, it remains manageable all the way through the cycle except during a brief period of planned overreaching, when they train close to their limit for a week or two before tapering and racing.

Fourth, the pros compete sparingly, aware that races are disruptive to the flow of training. They take a nice long break after the most important race to recharge their physical and emotional batteries.

Fifth and finally, the pros get the rest they need within the training cycle by reducing their training load every third or fourth week and by taking occasional days off from running.

Together, these planning guidelines represent a framework for your future training. But again, they are not a complete blueprint. Let's now begin the process of filling in this blueprint with the specifics of how to truly run like a pro by taking a deep dive into the question of *how much* you should run.

Coach's Tip

Adjusting Your Plan

In the preceding chapter, Matt gave you five rules that will help you begin designing your own training plan, and that's great. But a good training plan is worth little without good execution. To get the most out of your plan, you must make smart decisions about how to keep things on track when unforeseen circumstances arise. Much of what I know about proper training execution was learned the hard way when I coached myself between 2005 and 2006, and then again from 2008 to 2010. Here are my top three tips to help you avoid making the same mistakes I made.

1. DON'T OVERREACT TO ONE BAD WORKOUT.

I say this a lot, and I believe I can trace it back to 2005, when I was training for the US Marathon Championships, which were to be held in conjunction with the Twin Cities Marathon. My training segment, which I wrote in part with the help of my good friend Mike Nelson, had gone very well. Despite the heat and humidity in Saint Louis, I had crushed all my big marathon-specific workouts and was as fit as I had ever been. With ten days remaining before the race, I was supposed to knock out six miles at marathon pace. Nothing fancy—just a chance to feel the rhythm that I wanted to run in Minnesota. I even went to a track that night so I could be super exact about the splits.

It did not go well. I struggled from the first step. My legs felt like lead. I had to stop three miles in, and afterward I was an emotional wreck. The pace I wanted to run for 26.2 miles was too much for me over just three miles, and the race was less than two weeks away.

I lost it mentally and really freaked out. At twenty-five years old, I was too immature and too inexperienced to know how to handle it. I am ashamed to say it, but I basically gave up on the possibility that the race could be a success. In fact, that Sunday, one week before the marathon, I completed a medium-long run and then went straight downtown to the Saint Louis Rams football game, where I proceeded to tailgate (i.e., pound Budweisers) with my uncle and his buddies for about two hours before heading into the stadium for even more drinking during the three-hour game. Fifteen beers later, I was passed out on my couch, the Twin Cities Marathon the furthest thing from my mind.

Miraculously (or so it seemed at the time), I actually felt pretty darn good on my run the next day, and even better in my final work-out before the race: 2 x 3 miles at marathon pace. The pace that not even a week earlier I couldn't hit if my life depended on it now came easily—flowing out of me as if it were the pace I was put on this earth to run. Of course, I realize now that none of this was a miracle at all. It was simply the taper beginning to pay off. Based on years of anec-dotal evidence, I can tell you this phenomenon is quite common when dialing back the mileage two weeks before a marathon. The first week feels odd. The body has become used to doing a certain amount of work week in and week out, and when you take some of that work away, it rebels a bit. But that second week, things begin to come around. You get some pop back in your legs. Your energy level rises. All of that work you put in during the segment has now been absorbed and you are ready to unleash your fitness.

For me, that fitness was unleashed on the streets of Minneapolis and Saint Paul. I woke up on race day with a special feeling. All seemed right in the world. I took a bus to the starting area, where I did a short warm-up jog, and to this day, I cannot ever remember my legs feeling as good as they did that morning. Of course, the coach in me is obligated to remind you that it doesn't matter how you feel during your warm-up. You can feel terrible and then have a great

40

race. But feeling like a million bucks sure isn't a bad thing! It wasn't for me that day, anyway. I went on to finish second in the race and took home $20,500, which *also* felt like a million bucks, by far the largest payday I ever had as an athlete.

2. LISTEN TO YOUR BODY.

You would think the experience I just described would have taught me how to taper for a marathon. Nope. Part of the self-coaching process is learning from your mistakes. But you have to take the right lessons from those mistakes, not fit your findings to a self-affirming narrative. Coming off the success I had at Twin Cities in 2005, I picked the Grandma's Marathon in June 2006 as my next target. Having finished second at Twin Cities, I didn't think winning Grandma's was out of the question. My training that spring was off the charts. I was running the most mileage of my career, my workouts were faster than ever, and I set personal bests at two miles, four miles, and 10,000 meters during the segment. I felt invincible.

But as I approached the final few weeks of training, I made two huge mistakes. It started when my long-distance girlfriend, who lived in Portland, Oregon, decided to make the move to Saint Louis. For some reason we thought it would be a good idea for me to fly out to Oregon, load up her stuff, and drive all the way back with her—in the middle of a 120-mile week. (For the record, that girlfriend has since become my wife and the mother of my child, so no regrets. But I digress.)

The trip ended exactly two weeks before the race. I had reached the taper, but I had reached it exhausted—again. At this point, I ought to have said to myself, *Remember what happened last time, you idiot. Just back off, trust the taper, and you'll be fine.* Instead, because my (incorrect) analysis of what went wrong before Twin Cities was that I had tapered too much, I'd come into the Grandma's segment planning on running ninety miles two weeks before the race to avoid that crappy feeling I had endured ten days before Twin Cities. Of course, when I wrote the outline, I had not planned on a four-day

41

cross-country trip right before the taper was to begin. One of the golden rules of writing a training plan is to do so in pencil and allow for future adjustments.

I didn't. Utterly set in my conviction that a milder taper was the answer, I grinded through my ninety-mile week as scheduled. The workout I drew up for myself ten days out was even more challenging than the one I had tried and failed to do the previous fall: 3 x 2 miles at ten to fifteen seconds per mile faster than race pace with half-mile jog recoveries. I hit it, but I had to work really hard. And I paid for it during the medium-long run I did three days later, a run where you want to be cruising along and enjoying the distance, which I did not.

I backed off the mileage somewhat the week of the race, but no more than originally planned. My stubborn mind and body slogged through my standard final workout—2 x 3 miles at marathon pace— the same session that felt so glorious the previous fall, only this time it was a nightmare. I felt almost as bad as I had that evening eight months earlier when I had to step off the track after just three miles. I'd now had three subpar workouts in a row, and no time left to do anything about it before the race. I had dug myself into a hole.

As you can imagine, I woke up on race morning in Duluth a very different person than I had in Saint Paul the year before. I distinctly remember looking in the mirror and seeing bags under my eyes. On top of all of that, the weather was hot and muggy—nasty conditions, even if I'd done everything right. Surprise, surprise, my legs felt heavy from the get-go. Every mile felt harder than it should have. By halfway, I was already headed in the wrong direction. I finished in sixteenth place, more than thirteen minutes behind the winner and six minutes slower than I'd run at Twin Cities.

It took me a long time to get over that disappointment. In some ways, I never got over it with respect to the marathon. Not only was I soured mentally, but physically I could never again capture the sort of marathon-specific fitness I had that spring. I would go on to DNF (did not finish) the 2007 Houston Marathon, run poorly at the 2007 Boston Marathon, and finish nearly dead last at the 2008 US Olympic trials (held in the fall of 2007 in Central Park). For all intents and purposes, that was the end of my career as a marathoner.

Fear not, for I did run fast in other events and found a way to really enjoy my last couple of years of competitive running. But much of that enjoyment, and those successes, stemmed from the fact that I was never again as stubborn as I was during that Grandma's buildup. If my body was sluggish in consecutive workouts, I listened. If life stress was dampening my overall energy level, I listened. And, quite frankly, if I just didn't feel like running one day, I listened.

At the risk of sounding like Uncle Rico from *Napoleon Dynamite* who can't let go of the past, I must say that, had I only acknowledged those same signals before Grandma's, the race outcome might have been much different. A simple day off after the trip would have been a nice start. Seventy miles two weeks out instead of ninety would likely have changed things. And a revised race-week workout could have been the final piece. But alas, on that occasion, I did not listen.

3. IT'S (ALMOST) NEVER TOO LATE TO TURN THINGS AROUND.

But hey, if at first you don't succeed, try, try again. Eleven years after Grandma's, and long after my own career was dead and buried, I was once again faced with some tough decisions with a major race looming. Only this time it wasn't my race—it was Scott Smith's. Scott is an athlete I've coached on the NAZ Elite team since its inception in 2014. By the fall of 2017, I knew him pretty darn well. We had been through three marathons together and were preparing for the Frankfurt Marathon, where Scott would be taking a crack at recording a big personal best.

The training segment started off with all sorts of promise. Scott was training with teammates Scott Fauble and Matt Llano. The three of them had a nice rapport and the vibe was good. Scott and Scott (a.k.a. the Scotts) ran a very solid ten-mile race near the end of August. September got off to a good start, but then, out of the blue,

43

things began to unravel. Scott Smith had to stop ten miles into a fourteen-mile marathon-pace workout. The next session also came to an early halt. That was two bad workouts in a row. One bad workout does not a bad segment make. But two? That's a different story.

Without hesitation, I told Scott to take a day off. Then I gave him another easy day. We did some blood work to find out what might be wrong. Sure enough, his white blood cell count was high, indicating he was fighting off some sort of infection. So we pulled back on the intensity of his training. His next workout was supposed to be 10 x 1 mile at 4:45. We changed it to 4:55, and he hit it. That gave him some momentum. Scott had a pretty good marathon-pace workout right before leaving for Europe, two weeks before the race. When he got there, the snowball continued to roll in the right direction. I remember telling my wife, "Scott Smith's coming around." He felt good. Sure, he had missed some of the work as it was originally prescribed, but he had also nailed the vast majority.

At this point, it wasn't about squeezing things in. It was about being mentally and physically ready to go. On race day, he crushed it. His finish time of 2:12:21 was more than two minutes faster than his previous best, he took eighth place overall, and he was our top man on the day, ahead of both Scott and Matt, who by all accounts had had "better" training segments. As I now so often say, "It's about being ready on the day."

MATT FITZGERALD AND BEN ROSARIO

MANAGE MILEAGE
LIKE A PRO

ONE OF THE WORLD'S leading scientific experts on endurance training is Stephen Seiler, an American exercise physiologist who lives and works in Norway. Seiler is best known for his research on balancing different intensities in training, a topic we'll explore in the next chapter, but he's also produced some interesting work in other areas, including a somewhat whimsical yet useful infographic he dubbed "Seiler's Hierarchy of Endurance Training Needs."

The concept is borrowed from the influential psychologist Abraham Maslow, who developed a hierarchy of basic human needs in the 1940s—a five-tier pyramid that ranks our species' biological, psychological, and social needs in order of importance. Similarly, Seiler's hierarchy ranks eight widely practiced endurance-training methods in the order of their impact on fitness and performance. These rankings are based not just on experimental science but also on the real-world practices of elite athletes, with the most impactful method forming the foundation of the pyramid, the next most impactful method forming the second tier, and so on.

In Seiler's judgment, the most important factor in endurance training, occupying the ground floor of his pyramid, is "Frequency/Volume of Training." For runners, this means it's important—indeed, more important than anything else—to *run a lot*. And it explains why nearly all professional runners run twice a day most days and more than one hundred miles per week most weeks. As we've discussed, few nonelite runners can safely match these exact numbers, but the underlying principle of running a lot relative to one's individual limits applies to every runner. Let's address the question of why this is the case before moving on to some practical guidelines for how often and how much you run.

THE BENEFITS OF RUNNING A LOT

With any form of exercise, there exists what's known as a dose-response relationship between the amount of exercise done and the benefits that result from it. Take weight lifting, for example. If you're not currently lifting weights and want to get stronger, pumping iron for just five minutes three times a week will make you a little stronger. But if you're already doing that and want to get even stronger, you'll need to move up to a larger dose of weight lifting—say, fifteen minutes three times a week. And when you're ready, adding a fourth weekly session to your routine will provide an additional response.

A clear dose-response relationship exists with running as well. We saw a hint of this in chapter 1, where I described a couple of studies showing strong correlations between training volume and performance in large groups of runners. Further evidence of a dose-response relationship between training volume and running performance comes from a 2016 study published in *BMC Sports Science, Medicine and Rehabilitation*. Andrew Vickers and Emily Vertosick of the Memorial Sloan Kettering Cancer Center used an internet survey to collect training data and race times from more than 2,300 recreational runners. After crunching the numbers, they concluded that although "it is typically believed that training volume is more important for distances such as the marathon than for the 5 and 10 km distance. . . . [T]he association between training mileage and race velocity is similar across race distances."

It's no accident that the runners who train the most—the pros—are also the fastest runners. Obviously, talent plays a role as well. The typical one-hundred-plus-miles-per-week elite runner would still outperform the typical thirty-miles-per-week nonelite runner even if he cut his training volume by 70 percent. But he wouldn't race as fast as he does at higher volume. We know this because elite runners of past generations did run less, and they were slower. When Englishman Jim Peters set his fourth and final world record for the marathon in 1954, clocking 2:17:39 at the Polytechnic Marathon in London, he did so having averaged one hundred miles per week in training. When Eliud Kipchoge set the existing marathon world record of 2:01:39 in Berlin in 2018, he did so having averaged 120 miles per week in training—a full 20 percent more than Peters did. Elite training practices have certainly evolved in other ways since the 1950s, but greater volume is the biggest change.

Even among today's elite runners, those who run more tend to run better. This was shown in a study done by British and Spanish researchers and published in the *Journal of Strength and Conditioning Research* in 2019. The authors collected training and race performance data from a group of eighty-five elite male runners over a period of seven years, looking for training factors that contributed to better competitive results. What they found was that the amount of "easy" (i.e., low-intensity) running individual runners did was the single best predictor of how well they performed in competition.

Why low-intensity running in particular? The short answer is that there's only so much high-intensity running a runner can absorb, and indeed the extra twenty or so miles per week that today's pros are logging consist entirely of low-intensity work. I'll address the subject of intensity more fully in chapter 4. For now, suffice it to say that running a lot is good for performance. As to the question of why this is so, science tells us there are three major benefits of high-volume training: greater fitness, better efficiency, and heightened durability. Let's take a closer look at each of these.

Greater Fitness

Running fitness has many components, but none is more important than aerobic capacity (also known as VO_2max), or the ability to use inspired oxygen to power muscle contractions. An exceptionally high aerobic capacity is an absolute requirement for reaching the professional ranks as a distance runner. Both genetics and training contribute to aerobic capacity, and while much is made of the efficacy of high-intensity interval training in boosting VO_2max, high-volume training is even more effective. This is evidenced by the fact that elite athletes in all endurance disciplines who train at very high volume but with only a small fraction of their training at high intensity score much higher on VO_2max tests than elite athletes in sports like ice hockey and boxing, who typically do a lot less total cardiovascular training but with greater emphasis on high intensity.

Running is not the only endurance sport in which longitudinal increases in training volume have yielded higher levels of fitness and performance at the elite stratum. The same thing happened in rowing, and in 2004, Stephen Seiler got together with Åke Fiskerstrand of the Norwegian Rowing Federation to quantify this evolution. What they found was that, between 1971 and 2000, average training volume in elite rowers increased by 20 percent, while VO_2max scores increased by 12 percent and average power output in a six-minute rowing ergometer test grew by 10 percent. To be clear, even in 1971 elite rowers were training at high volumes, but as time passed and elite rowers of succeeding generations trained at even higher volumes, they became fitter and faster. Now, running is not rowing, of course, but performance is equally dependent on aerobic capacity in both sports, so it's no stretch to generalize these findings to encompass all major endurance disciplines, running included.

Exactly how high-volume training contributes to maximizing aerobic capacity is not yet fully understood, but it may have to do with a phenomenon known as glycogen flux. Glycogen is the storage form of carbohydrate in the body, and it is a critical source of energy for running—intense running in particular. When glycogen stores deplete through training, genes involved in boosting aerobic capacity become more active. Subsequent rest and carbohydrate intake then replenish these fuel stores, preparing the athlete to deplete them again. The more flux a runner experiences in her glycogen stores over time, the more she stimulates her genes to boost her aerobic capacity, and no runner experiences more glycogen flux than one who eats plenty of carbs, rests adequately, *and runs a lot*, as the pros do.

Another component of running fitness that can only be maximized through high-volume training is endurance. Also referred to as fatigue resistance, endurance is truly the name of the game in any race longer than a sprint. Whether you're a miler, an ultrarunner, or anything in between, your goal is not to get faster, per se, but to run at higher and higher percentages of your top speed for longer and longer periods of time before fatigue forces you to slow down.

Arthur Lydiard's most successful athlete, Peter Snell, won three Olympic gold medals at 800 and 1500 meters in the early 1960s on a regimen of ninety- to one-hundred-mile weeks that was unheard of at the time for middle-distance runners. The coach explained the rationale in a 1962 *Sports Illustrated* essay titled "Why I Prescribe Marathons for Milers." "In theory," he wrote, "I am trying to develop my runners until they are in a tireless state. In practice, this means I am trying to give them sufficient stamina to maintain their natural speed over whatever distance they are running. Stamina is the key to the whole thing, because you can take speed for granted. No? Look here. Everybody thinks a four-minute mile is terrific, but it is only four one-minute quarter miles. Practically any athlete can run one one-minute quarter, but few have the stamina to run four of them in a row. How do you give them the necessary stamina? By making them run and run and run some more."

It took a while, but science has since provided empirical validation of Lydiard's observation. Some of this evidence comes from that huge study involving training data from fourteen thousand runners I described in chapter 1. For the purposes of their research, collaborators Thorsten Emig and Jussi Peltonen defined endurance as the percentage of an individual runner's VO_2max they could sustain for one hour. By this definition, a runner can increase their endurance and performance without getting faster in any pure sense by increasing the percentage of their VO_2max they can sustain for one hour—a concept that is analogous to Lydiard's notion of stamina. The data that Emig and Peltonen collected from their subjects showed that relatively modest improvements in endurance translated to large improvements in race times, and that higher training volumes were closely linked to better endurance.

49

Better Efficiency

Fitness isn't the only factor that contributes to running performance. Running is also a *skill*. There are elite cyclists and rowers and cross-country skiers whose VO_2max scores match that of any pro runner, and yet they could never run as well. Having a high aerobic capacity enables an athlete to sustain high levels of energy output, which translates to the ability to go fast for an extended period of time. Running *skill* minimizes the amount of effort it takes a runner to run, enabling them to go faster and longer at any level of fitness.

How do you become a more skillful runner? The same way you become a more skillful juggler: practice. Throughout every run you do, your brain is in constant communication with proprioceptive nerves in every part of your body, looking for ways to trim waste from the motor program it uses for running. This process is unconscious, automatic, and highly effective. In a 2007 study published in the *European Journal of Applied Physiology*, Iain Hunter and Gerald Smith of the Norwegian School of Sport Sciences measured changes in the stride rate and stride frequency of runners over the course of a one-hour treadmill time trial. What they discovered was that these changes, which happened unconsciously, served to minimize the loss of efficiency that naturally occurs as a runner fatigues. Without even knowing it, these runners subtly adjusted the way they ran within a single run to save energy.

But wait—it gets better. There's evidence that, although this process does slow down over time, it never peters out entirely. In a 2011 study, researchers at the University of New Hampshire compared various fitness measures as well as running economy (which you can think of as the running equivalent of fuel efficiency) in runners representing three different age ranges: eighteen to thirty-nine, forty to fifty-nine, and over sixty. Unsurprisingly, they found that VO_2max, maximal heart rate, speed, strength, and power declined with age. But running economy did not, which is rather curious, because muscle strength and power are important contributors to running economy. The fact that the oldest runners were no less economical than

50

their younger counterparts despite these losses suggests that, on a neuromotor level, they were actually *more* efficient.

This is good news for runners who take the long view, as it allows them to look forward to getting better and better at the skill of running. But it may be bad news for those who are in a hurry to become more skillful. By its very nature, experience takes time to accumulate. You can accelerate the process to some extent, however, by running a lot, and indeed the aforementioned Emig–Peltonen study found that the positive relationship between training mileage and race performance was mediated primarily by gains in running economy. This particular finding helps explain why elite runners routinely produce their best race times in their thirties despite recording their highest VO_2max readings in their early twenties.

Heightened Durability

Running is associated with a variety of overuse injuries such as plantar fasciitis, shin splints, and patellofemoral pain. You might assume that because running is causally related to these injuries, the more a person runs, the more likely they are to get injured. In fact, almost the opposite is true.

A 2013 study by Danish researchers found that, among 662 runners training for a marathon, those who ran less than thirty kilometers per week were injured more than twice as often as those who ran thirty to sixty kilometers per week, while those who ran more than sixty kilometers per week were no more likely to get injured than those who ran between thirty and sixty kilometers. One year later, a similar study published in the *Journal of Science and Medicine and Sport* reported that, within a group of 517 recreational runners, those who ran the least were injured the most. And a 2016 study by Dutch scientists found that even within a group of newer runners, those who did the least running had the most injuries.

Why do runners who run more get injured less? There are two main reasons. One is that running stimulates tissue adaptations in the bones, muscles, and joints that make these structures more durable, hence more resistant to injury. Think about it: Who is more likely to get injured during a ten-mile run—a runner who *routinely* runs ten miles or one who has *never* run that far? The answer is obvious. The runner who routinely runs ten miles will have adapted to the stress of pounding out this distance to a degree the other runner hasn't.

In short, running protects against the very injuries it sometimes causes. The stress of running inflicts microscopic damage on the tissues of the lower extremities. If the next stress-imposing run comes too quickly, this damage accumulates and becomes an injury. If not, the healing process leaves the tissues stronger than they were before, hence more resistant to future damage. It's when the muscles, bones, and connective tissues are exposed to more stress than they're ready for that breakdowns occur, and only running can prepare these tissues for the stress of running.

This was shown in a study conducted by Mitchell Rauh at San Diego State University and published in the *Journal of Orthopaedic & Sports Physical Therapy* in 2014. Rauh tracked injuries in a group of 421 high school runners over the course of a fall cross country season and found that those who spent fewer than eight weeks running during the preceding summer were far more likely to get injured than were those who ran eight weeks or more. The athletes who had taken the time to get their legs ready for it better tolerated the rigors of in-season training and racing.

Even runners who routinely run a lot are at risk of getting injured when they increase their mileage too abruptly, as was demonstrated in a 2020 study published in *International Journal of Sports Medicine*. A team of Dutch and German researchers enlisted twenty-three recreational runners to keep detailed training diaries for two years. The data showed that anytime their acute training load (the combined volume and intensity of their training over the past week) exceeded their chronic training load (the combined volume and intensity of their training over the past four weeks) by more than 10 percent, the likelihood of an injury occurring within the next two to three weeks spiked. The take-home lesson here is simply this: the best way to manipulate your running mileage if you wish to minimize injury risk is to gradually build up to a high volume of running and then keep it there.

The other reason runners who run more get injured less is that running more leads to changes in running form that reduce stress on the lower extremities. Earlier in the chapter, we saw that running a lot causes changes in biomechanics that make the stride more efficient. It turns out these same changes also reduce injury risk. In another 2014 study, researchers at the University of Massachusetts Amherst analyzed the biomechanics of "low-mileage" (less than fifteen miles per week) and "high-mileage" (more than twenty miles per week) runners and were able to identify several differences between the two groups that, they wrote, "may explain the lower incidence of overuse knee injuries for higher mileage runners."

By no means am I suggesting that "more is better" in an absolute sense. If that were the case, the pros would run even more than they do. But what the evidence clearly does show is that running a lot is far less risky than many runners assume.

HOW MUCH SHOULD YOU RUN?

For the vast majority of nonelite runners, training volume is limited not by physical factors but by psychological, social, and lifestyle factors. As we saw in chapter 1, runners who don't race for a living commonly settle into a particular level of training either because they don't feel they're "good enough" to run more or because their peers run the same amount, or both. But even when these factors aren't at play, career and family responsibilities often won't permit a runner to spend more time training, or the runner may simply have no desire to.

I respect every runner's right to set his own limit on running mileage. My goal here is simply to offer guidelines on how to manage your mileage for maximum performance, as the pros do. If you follow these guidelines and still choose to limit your training volume to a comfortable level that is below your physical limit, I'm confident you'll be happy with both your running performance and your overall life balance.

Go from Zero to Seven—Slowly

Let's assume you're new to running—an absolute beginner. And let's further assume that you haven't been exercising much at all recently, you could stand to lose a few pounds, and you're not a spring chicken. How the heck are *you* supposed to emulate the pros, mileage-wise?

Keep in mind, every pro runner was a beginner once too. There's a proven process for earning the benefits of running a lot, and though each runner has a different starting point, the process is generally the same for all. For the person who is truly at square one, it's best to begin with a schedule of alternate-day running. When you're just starting off, you need to give your body a full forty-eight hours to recover from and adapt to the tissue disruptions imposed by each run before attempting the next one. And your runs shouldn't be pure running either, but alternating segments of walking and slow jogging. At first, the run segments should be quite short. If all goes well, you can lengthen these segments gradually over a period of several weeks until you're able to run for thirty minutes straight. Table 3.1 shows a suggested four-week program for a raw beginner.

• TABLE 3.1 •
SUGGESTED TRAINING PROGRAM FOR NEW RUNNERS

Week 1	15 x (1:00 walk/1:00 jog)	Rest or Cross-Training	15 x (1:00 walk/1:00 jog)	Rest or Cross-Training	10 x (1:00 walk/2:00 jog)	Rest or Cross-Training	10 x (1:00 walk/2:00 jog)
Week 2	Rest or Cross-Training	8 x (1:00 walk/3:00 jog)	Rest or Cross-Training	8 x (1:00 walk/3:00 jog)	Rest or Cross-Training	6 x (1:00 walk/4:00 jog)	Rest or Cross-Training
Week 3	6 x (1:00 walk/4:00 jog)	Rest or Cross-Training	5 x (1:00 walk/5:00 jog)	Rest or Cross-Training	5 x (1:00 walk/5:00 jog)	Rest or Cross-Training	3 x (1:00 walk/9:00 jog)
Week 4	Rest or Cross-Training	3 x (1:00 walk / 9:00 jog)	Rest or Cross-Training	2 x (1:00 walk/14:00 jog)	Rest or Cross-Training	30:00 jog	Rest or Cross-Training

54

As you see, the program includes optional cross-training sessions on nonrunning days. Exercising this option one or more times each week will accelerate your fitness development in a way that doesn't interfere with your main goal of avoiding injury as you build up a tolerance for running. Your cross-training may take the form of strength training yoga, Pilates, or nonimpact cardio exercise such as bicycling (we'll come back to nonimpact cardio later in the chapter).

Okay, so you've gotten to the point where you can run for thirty minutes straight every other day without getting hurt. Now what? Set your sights on the Seven-Hour Standard. This is my name for the level of running volume I advise every performance-seeking runner to aspire to. The Seven-Hour Standard is doing seven hours of running per week distributed across either six days with one day of absolute rest or seven days with one day of relative rest.

Why seven hours? A few reasons. First, if you have time to run on a given day, you probably have time for a one-hour run. Second, your lifestyle probably allows you to run most days, if not every day. Add these two things together and you get seven hours of weekly running. And you can do *a lot* with this amount of training if you make good use of the time—far more than you could with less training.

Naturally, you can achieve even more with even greater amounts of running. But that comes later, and only for those whose physical capacity, motivation, and lifestyle permit further increases. What matters for the newer runner is attaining the Seven-Hour Standard safely, a process that is simply an extension of the stepwise progression shown in Table 3.1.

Once you're able to run for thirty minutes a day every other day, try running on consecutive days once a week and see how that goes. If you survive a month of four runs per week, add a fifth, and so on. Feel free to add duration to some of these runs, as well—in small increments, of course—slowly moving closer to the Seven-Hour Standard in terms of both running frequency and average run duration until you get there.

Measure by Time, Not by Distance

You may have noticed that in the previous section I offered time-based guidelines for increasing running volume, whereas previously I referred mainly to distance. The truth of the matter is that, although most runners prefer to measure their training in miles or kilometers, it's actually better to regulate volume by time. The reason is that the amount of stress that running imposes on the body is determined by time exposure, not by distance covered.

A quick example will help you understand why. The term *velocity at VO$_2$max* (vVO$_2$max) denotes the lowest speed at which an individual runner reaches her maximal rate of oxygen consumption and which, for runners of all abilities, equates to the fastest speed that can be sustained for about six minutes. Whether you are a total beginner, an Olympian, or anything in between, you'll reach exhaustion after running at your personal vVO$_2$max for six minutes or thereabouts. The difference is that, whereas a beginner might cover less than 0.75 mile in those six minutes, an elite female runner will cover 1.25 miles, and a male pro nearly 1.5 miles. Thus, if you're a coach who wants to design a workout targeting vVO$_2$max that is equally challenging for both a novice runner and an elite runner, you need to make the workout time-based rather than distance-based.

The same principle applies to weekly training volume. A typical pro runner spends about twelve hours per week running, give or take. But because the typical pro runner is very fast, he covers 110 to 120 miles in that time. A well-trained nonelite runner who wants to train just as hard as the pros will achieve his objective not by matching this distance but by matching the time, and covering "only" sixty-five to seventy miles per week.

If you prefer to continue to measure your training by distance, that's okay. The pros do too. Just bear in mind that your body measures things in time.

Find Your Level

Let's suppose now that you want to go all the way with your running—to find out how good you can be with an absolute commitment to the sport, just like the pros. In that case, you'll probably want to go beyond the Seven-Hour Standard in your running volume. But understand that the goal is not to keep running more and more until you hit the ultimate limit of your body's tolerance. Rather, it's to keep running more until you discover the amount of running that gives you the best results in terms of fitness and performance. There is a difference between the maximal amount of running you can possibly handle and the amount of running that is maximally beneficial. I refer to the latter quantity as a runner's mileage sweet spot.

There are two ways to increase your running volume beyond the Seven-Hour Standard: extend the runs you're already doing, and run more frequently. Generally speaking, running more frequently is slightly gentler on the body than increasing volume by an equal amount through extending your existing runs. This is why the pros distribute their ten to fifteen hours of weekly running across twelve or thirteen separate runs instead of just six or seven.

Seven hours per week is close to the maximum amount of running you'll want to do on a routine basis before you begin to consider doubling—i.e., running twice—on some days. This may seem like a big step if you've never done it before, but it's really just a matter of dividing the total volume of running you're likely to do anyway into more and smaller parts (and, yes, having to do laundry slightly more often).

In your search for your personal mileage sweet spot, I encourage you to focus less on achieving a certain weekly mileage total and more on finding a stable weekly training structure that seems to yield optimal results. In theory, there are dozens of possible structures you could adopt, but in practice, coaches have found that a handful of routines tend to work best for the vast majority of improvement-seeking runners who are willing and able to set their volume ceiling at least as high as the Seven-Hour Standard. These are shown in Table 3.2.

· TABLE 3.2 ·

PROVEN WEEKLY TRAINING STRUCTURES

OPTION A—SIX TO SEVEN RUNS PER WEEK

Easy Run or Day Off	Hard Run	Easy Run	Easy Run	Hard Run	Easy Run	Long/Hard Run

OPTION B—NINE RUNS PER WEEK

A.M.	Easy Run	Hard Run	Easy Run	Easy Run	Hard Run	Easy Run	Long/Hard Run
P.M.		Easy Run			Easy Run		

OPTION C—TWELVE RUNS PER WEEK

A.M.	Easy Run	Hard Run	Easy Run	Easy Run	Hard Run	Easy Run	Long/Hard Run
P.M.		Easy Run	Easy Run	Easy Run	Easy Run	Easy Run	

Climb the ladder of these weekly training structures one rung at a time. If you're currently hovering around six runs and seven hours per week, try seven runs. If you don't see improvement, or if at this training frequency you experience indicators that you are at or near your limit (incipient injuries, mounting fatigue, poor workouts), drop back to six runs. If you see improvement and experience only small setbacks (such as normal aches and pains) at a frequency you can live with, you've found your sweet spot. And if you see improvement and are able to manage the training load fairly comfortably, consider advancing to option B and repeat the same evaluative process.

Once you've found your optimal weekly training structure, feel free to fine-tune your training volume within it. Don't assume that choosing any particular routine locks you into a fixed mileage. For example, you could choose option C and make your second runs really short, as I myself did when I first tried doubling on a regular basis. Two easy miles in the afternoon five times per week didn't seem like much on paper, but I was thankful for those few extra miles of training when I ran my next marathon!

CONSIDER YOUR EVENT FOCUS,
BUT NOT TOO MUCH

In principle, your optimal weekly mileage in training for shorter races such as 5Ks is likely to be lower than your optimal weekly mileage in training for longer events such as marathons. This is because you are (or should be) doing a greater percentage of your training at high intensity in 5K training, which limits the total running volume you can handle, and also because your longest runs need not be as long in 5K training.

At the professional level, athletes focused on middle-distance track events typically run a lot less than athletes focused on longer road or trail events. But this doesn't necessarily mean you should run a lot less when you're training for a short race than you do when training for a longer one. That's because most nonelite runners don't run enough to maximize their performance in races of *any* distance, including shorter ones.

Have you ever noticed that runners often set personal bests at shorter distances when they're in the midst of training for longer events? The reason is that only when they are training for longer distances do most nonelite runners run enough to perform at their best in shorter races. And have you ever noticed how those online race time predictors tend to be pretty good at predicting (for example) the time you could run a 10K based on a recent 5K performance, but they tend to overestimate marathon performance based on times for shorter distances? It's not that the calculators are faulty. It's that very seldom are nonelite runners as well prepared for marathons, volume-wise, as they are for shorter events.

There is a pretty good chance that the maximum amount of running you're either physically able to do or willing to do is not greater than the amount that will optimize your results in shorter races. If this is indeed the case, and if you like to compete at a range of distances, then my advice for you is that you remain open to training about as much for shorter races as you do for longer ones. Choosing a weekly training structure that you use for all race distances will help encourage this kind of consistency. And speaking of consistency . . .

59

Be Consistent, but Not Too Consistent

As I mentioned earlier in the chapter, overuse injuries are most likely to occur when the training load is increasing—that is, when you're adding volume, intensity, or both to your training. For this reason, it's best to aim for consistency in your training volume. But there is such a thing as too much consistency.

If you consistently train close to your physical ceiling in running volume, your chances of getting injured are very high. Runners are more likely to get injured when they're testing their limits. This happens not only when a runner is running more and more in an effort to increase their limit but also when a runner has found his ultimate limit and tries to stay near it too long. Running more and more is not inherently risky, nor is running a lot. These things are only risky when they entail testing limits, and when they don't, they're safe. For example, after dropping out of the 2018 Boston Marathon with hypothermia and deciding to try again at Grandma's Marathon eight weeks later, NAZ Elite member Kellyn Taylor took a week off from running, then ran forty-two miles the next week, seventy-nine miles the week after that, and ninety-seven miles the week after that. It sounds risky but it wasn't, because Kellyn had peaked at 128 miles just a few weeks earlier, in her buildup to Boston, so although she was increasing her mileage rather aggressively and running a lot, she wasn't really testing her limit.

When it is said of a given pro runner that she runs x miles per week, this does not mean she runs x miles *every* week. More likely, this number represents her peak volume, or something close to it. And as we've discussed, peaks are not sustainable for long periods. What *is* sustainable for every runner is an amount of running that's slightly lower than their current ceiling, and that's the volume level you'll want to hang out near at most times. If you fall too far below it for too long, you'll face a high risk of injury in getting back there, and if you stray too far above it for too long, you'll face a high risk of both injury and burnout as a result of continuously testing your limit. Including regular recovery weeks in your training, where you intentionally buck the general trend of mileage increase, is another way to mitigate these risks without eschewing the inherently somewhat risky work that is required to attain peak race fitness.

Let's put some numbers on this guidance. Suppose you like to do half marathons, and experience has taught you it's best not to go above sixty miles in your heaviest weeks of training for this distance. In this case, a median mileage in the range of forty-five to fifty miles per week will probably serve you well. Over the course of a full year, you should be within this range in the majority of weeks, yet with continuous gentle fluctuations between low points marked by short breaks from formal training and brief high points right at that sixty-mile limit.

Consider Cross-Training

Some runners are naturally more injury-prone than others. Research indicates that certain unchangeable factors, including characteristics of joint collagen, make runners more susceptible to overuse injuries. If you're among those who drew this genetic short straw, you might be frustrated by an inability to consistently run as much as you'd like to without breaking down. In this case, you might want to consider padding your schedule with some cardiovascular cross-training in a low- or nonimpact modality such as bicycling. This will allow you to gain the lion's share of the fitness benefits associated with running more with less injury risk. That's right: cross-training isn't just for beginners!

Research proves it. In a 1998 study, Mick Flynn and colleagues at Purdue University added either three extra runs or three stationary bike workouts to the training programs of twenty runners for a period of six weeks. All the runners completed a five-kilometer time trial before this period of modified training and again afterward. Both the running-only group and the cross-training program improved their times by an average of 2.5 percent.

Additional proof of the effectiveness of cross-training comes from the real world. Many injury-prone pro runners have used cross-training to achieve performances they couldn't have achieved without it. Among them is Meb Keflezighi, winner of the 2009 New York City

Marathon and the 2014 Boston Marathon, who after suffering a calf injury in 2013 replaced his afternoon runs with outdoor elliptical biking and came back to take second place in the USATF Half Marathon Championships with a time of 1:01:22—at age thirty-eight!

The best cross-training activities for runners are those that closely simulate running but without the impact. These include indoor and outdoor bicycling, elliptical running, uphill treadmill walking, cross-country skiing, and Meb's choice, outdoor elliptical biking.

DON'T BE A SLAVE TO NUMBERS

Many years ago, I injured myself trying to complete my first one-hundred-mile week of running. Ignoring evidence that my personal sweet spot was in the high eighties to low nineties, I allowed myself to get caught up in the allure of crossing the triple-digit threshold, and I paid a price for it. It was a dumb mistake, but I am hardly the only runner to have sabotaged himself by becoming a slave to numbers. Whether it's twenty kilometers in a day or forty miles for a week or whatever, runners routinely land themselves in trouble by setting their heart on reaching a certain round number and ignoring warnings from their body that forcing it is not a good idea.

Elite coach Jerry Schumacher helps his athletes avoid this pitfall by having them measure their training volume in "Badger miles," which originated during Schumacher's time at the University of Wisconsin and are really just a backdoor way of measuring in time rather than distance (a Badger mile equals seven minutes). Many top East African runners avoid the same pitfall by not tracking weekly volume at all. They just take each day as it comes, basing today's mileage on where they are in the training process and on how they feel.

Your focus should be the same. I wouldn't go so far as to advise you not to even bother tracking your weekly training volume, as doing so can be useful in finding and staying in your sweet spot. But your main priority should be doing the right amount of running each day, letting the total take care of itself.

Discovering Your
Mileage Sweet Spot

Mileage is an often polarizing topic in our sport. But it doesn't have to be. As with many of the aspects of training that we cover in this book, figuring out your optimal weekly mileage is easier than some make it out to be. Let me take a crack at describing my philosophy in three bullet points:

- The best way to get better at running is to run.
- Exactly how much you ought to run depends on your life schedule, your biomechanical limitations, and your training history.
- Thus, weekly mileage becomes a moving target over time, but at any given point what we're trying to do is find the mileage at which we can maintain a healthy work/life balance, avoid injury, and properly execute our hard workouts.

These principles apply every bit as much to the pros I work with as they do to you. You might not know it, but there is actually a lot of variance in mileage among professional distance runners. Like you, the pros have to figure out the weekly mileage that is right for them. Also like you, they have a life, and biomechanical limitations, and key workouts that they need to hit.

We have athletes on our team, like Lauren Paquette, who run sixty-five to seventy miles per week; we have athletes, including Scott Fauble, who run 100 to 110 miles per week; and we even have athletes who have trained consistently at 110 to 120 miles per week, like Scott Smith. In Lauren's case, her relatively low mileage is not a work/life balance issue—she's a professional runner with plenty of time to recover. It's a biomechanical limitation. Lauren is a forefoot runner who puts a lot of pressure on her metatarsals, as well as on the surrounding muscles and tendons, with each and every stride she takes. It would be very risky for an athlete with that type of foot strike to run one-hundred-plus miles per week, in my opinion. Scott Fauble, on the other hand, has a very efficient foot strike for a distance runner and is a very strong athlete overall. Yet, for whatever reason, we have found over time that if we push the mileage too high, he struggles to execute the bigger workouts the way he wants to. Thus, we tend to keep him between 100 and 110 miles. Contrast him with his pal Scott Smith, who somehow seems to work out better when his mileage is at its highest.

Looking back on my own running career (if you want to call it that) also helps me. My own mileage trajectory was pretty standard for a male who starts running seriously in high school. My coach eased me into running more. As a freshman, I ran twenty to thirty miles per week. In my sophomore year, that number grew to thirty to forty miles. As a junior, I was consistently logging fifty to sixty miles per week, and as a senior, I hit the sixty to seventy range.

In college, my weekly mileage continued to climb, though it never got above eighty to ninety on any consistent basis. After college, I jumped up above one hundred miles per week, and from there to 120 fairly quickly. For the next five years, from age twenty-three to age twenty-seven, I averaged more than one hundred miles per week including brief breaks after competitive seasons.

I was fortunate. I could handle a lot of work and I did not have much in the way of biomechanical limitations. By the time I was twenty-seven, I had started my running specialty store in Saint Louis. My business partner and I were putting in sixty-hour workweeks on the regular. Life was one big stressful whirlwind. Needless to say, running one-hundred-mile weeks was becoming less and less feasible. So, after I competed in the 2008 US Olympic Trials Marathon, I decided my days of high mileage were over. In fact, I decided my days of competing at a high level were over, because I thought if you weren't running more than one hundred miles a week, you couldn't really expect to race at the level I had become accustomed to. But I was wrong.

I decided to take a totally new approach to my training. I no longer cared about my weekly mileage total, a stat I had obsessed over for years. I did write myself a training schedule, but if I missed a day, I didn't let it bother me. I took out most of my doubles, I reduced my weekly long run from twenty miles to fourteen, and while I kept up with doing one or two hard workouts per week, the total volume in those sessions dropped from ten to twelve miles of hard work to four to six miles, and sometimes even less.

That sort of training wasn't going to be conducive to running my personal best in the marathon. I knew that. So I didn't even try. But I figured maybe, just maybe, it could lead to fast times at some shorter distances. Lo and behold, it did—I ended up running a lifetime best mile of 4:03 at the age of twenty-nine. This from a guy who had only run the equivalent of a 4:19 in college. As I look back at all the races I've ever run, that 4:03 mile remains one of my absolute favorites (indeed, you haven't heard the last of it in this book!). And it would never have happened if I hadn't allowed myself to finally take my work/life balance into consideration when approaching my mileage.

The lesson I learned and wish to pass on to you is that weekly mileage is personal. There's no online algorithm that will, based on a few bits of input, tell you the exact right amount of running to do. This is something you must discover for yourself over time via classic trial and error, and it can, and should, be adjusted at various points in your running life. The ultimate goal, as we know from the pros, is to find your personal "sweet spot," as Matt calls it—yours and yours alone.

4

BALANCE INTENSITIES LIKE A PRO

*I*N 2010, SCIENTISTS FROM two Norwegian universities teamed up to study the training methods of their country's top runners. Six athletes agreed to participate, each of them submitting a year's worth of training data for analysis. Of the six, half were track specialists focused on events ranging from 3000 to 10,000 meters and the other half were road racers focused on the half-marathon and marathon distances. Of particular interest to the researchers were the volume and the intensity distribution of their training. We addressed volume in the preceding chapter, so let's concentrate on what was observed on the intensity side.

Between November and February (the "preparation period"), the three track athletes were found to have completed 76.4 percent of their running at low intensity (which is defined as anything done below 82 percent of maximum heart rate, a number that sounds arbitrary but is not, as you'll see presently). In March and April ("pre-competition period"), the same runners did 79 percent of their running at low intensity. And from May to August ("competition season"), they did 80.8 percent of their running at low intensity.

The road racers, despite competing at significantly greater distances, also hewed close to an 80 percent low / 20 percent moderate-to-high intensity balance throughout the year, completing 83.6, 84.7, and 79.9 percent of their running below 82 percent of maximum heart rate during the same three periods. In a paper published in the *Inter-*

national *Journal of Sports Science & Coaching*, the researchers concluded, "The main finding in this study . . . was that a relatively high training volume at low intensity . . . was beneficial for the development of running performance in six Norwegian male and female track and marathon runners competing at [the] top European level."

The consistent 80/20 intensity balance noted in this group of world-class runners is by no means unusual. A number of other studies have yielded similar findings. In 2003, for example, French exercise physiologist Véronique Billat reported that elite Kenyan runners did about 85 percent of their training below the lactate threshold, the intensity at which lactate, an intermediate product of aerobic metabolism, begins to accumulate in the blood, and which falls between 85 and 90 percent of maximum heart rate in the fittest athletes. Further, a 2012 analysis of the training of three top Canadian marathoners found that they completed 74 percent of their running at low intensity over the course of a season.

It doesn't stop there. Not only do elite runners all around the world adhere to an 80/20 intensity balance, but elite athletes in other endurance disciplines, including cross-country skiing, cycling, rowing, swimming, and triathlon, do as well. Take cyclists, for example. A 2017 study led by Dajo Sanders of Maastricht University reported that, over a ten-week period, professional cyclists spent 79.5 percent of their training time at low intensity (as measured by power output) and the remaining 20.5 percent at moderate and high intensities.

What makes this pattern even more intriguing is that it didn't always exist. Historical data reveals that the 80/20 intensity balance elite endurance athletes practice universally today was not widely practiced in *any* sport before the 1960s. Over a period of several decades, elite runners, rowers, cross-country skiers, and others gradually converged on this particular distribution of training intensities. Scientists refer to this type of process as *self-organization*. In nature, whenever a single, optimal solution exists to a particular problem, it is likely to be discovered independently in multiple populations. The so-called camera eye, an organ that, according to biologists, evolved independently in more than fifty species, is an often-cited example. In the case of endurance training, an 80/20 intensity balance appears to be optimal for fitness

67

and performance, and that's why top athletes in every major discipline and in all parts of the world hit upon it separately.

Remember Stephen Seiler, the scientist who gave us Seiler's Hierarchy of Endurance Training Needs? In a 2009 paper published in *Sportscience*, Seiler and coauthor Espen Tønnessen wrote, "In today's performance environment, where promising athletes have essentially unlimited time to train, all athletes train a lot and are highly motivated to optimize the training process. Training ideas that sound good but don't work in practice will fade away. Given these conditions . . . any consistent pattern of training intensity distribution emerging across sport disciplines is likely to be a result of a successful self-organization (evolution) towards a population optimum . . . an approach to training organization that results in most athletes staying healthy, making good progress, and performing well in their most important events."

Perhaps the most compelling proof that the 80/20 intensity balance is truly optimal in running is the fact that its use has made the world's best runners even better. One of the last great runners to come along before the 80/20 method took over the sport was Vladimir Kuts, who won Olympic gold for the Soviet Union at 5000 and 10,000 meters in 1956. Under coach Grigory Nikiforov, Kuts maintained a punishing training regimen that was heavy on high-intensity intervals. While it produced world records of 13:35.0 and 28:30.4 at the aforementioned distances, it may also have contributed to his untimely death at age forty-eight. In comparison, it is not uncommon for college runners today—all adhering to a more sustainable 80/20 balance—to surpass Kuts's times.

As compelling as it is, such real-world evidence of the superiority of the 80/20 approach says nothing about *why* it works better. Fortunately, we have science to satisfy our curiosity on this point.

MAXIMALLY EFFECTIVE DOSES

We've all heard the tongue-in-cheek phrase "If a little is good, more must be better." In fact, with few exceptions, the opposite is true—and high-intensity running is not among the exceptions. There's no denying that small amounts of high-intensity exercise increase fitness more than small amounts of low-intensity exercise—this has been shown in study after study. But the reason small amounts of high-intensity running yield significant fitness benefits is that they impose a lot of stress on the body, and for the very same reason, large amounts are increasingly harmful.

Studies prove this as well. In a 1999 experiment, French researchers had a small group of elite middle-distance runners run six times per week for twelve weeks. During the first four weeks, all six runs were done at low intensity. During the next four weeks, the runners did five runs at low intensity and one run at high intensity (an approximate 80/20 balance). Finally, during the last four weeks, they did three runs at low intensity and three at high intensity. After each four-week block, the runners completed a VO_2max test to measure changes in their aerobic capacity. On average, VO_2max scores were highest after the four-week block of 80/20 training, while the last block, focused on high intensity, produced the lowest scores. Notably, during the concluding four-week period, the runners also exhibited heightened levels of the stress hormone norepinephrine along with suppressed heart rates while running—two classic markers of nonfunctional overreaching.

With low intensity, it's a completely different story. Because it is less stressful to the body, low-intensity running yields small benefits when done in small amounts. But the relative gentleness of low-intensity running enables most runners to handle quite a lot of it, and the more we do (up to a point, naturally), the fitter we get.

A certain concept borrowed from the field of pharmacology (of all things) can help us make sense of all this. The term *maximally effective dose* refers to the specific dosage of a particular medicine that provides the most benefit to a patient. Almost always, this amount is greater than the *minimum effective dose* (the smallest amount that provides a measurable benefit) and less than the *maximum tolerable dose* (the largest amount that doesn't do more harm than good). For runners, the maximally effective dose of low-intensity training is far greater than the maximally effective dose of moderate-to-high-intensity training. This, in essence, is why the optimal balance of low and moderate-to-high intensity is 80/20, even though, minute for minute, high intensity is more effective.

You may be curious as to why I keep lumping together moderate and high intensity. An answer to this question—as well as to the question of how, exactly, moderate and high intensities are both more stressful than low—comes from a study led by our friend Stephen Seiler and published in *Medicine & Science in Sports & Exercise* in 2007. Seiler's team used a measure known as heart rate variability (HRV) to track the rate of autonomic nervous system recovery following bouts of exercise performed at a range of intensities by a mixed group of elite runners and fit young nonathletes. Seiler's team found that recovery was markedly slower after exercise at any intensity exceeding the *first ventilatory threshold (VT$_1$)*, which is the lower of two distinct exercise intensities at which the rate of oxygen consumption abruptly spikes. When the VT$_1$ is exceeded, the brain is forced to activate oxygen-hogging fast-twitch muscle fibers to generate the desired level of work output (specifically speed in the case of running). The brain itself has to work a lot harder when the body is working above the first ventilatory threshold, and this is what makes exercising even slightly above it more stressful than exercising just below it, resulting in longer recovery times and a lower maximum tolerable dose.

Since the birth of modern exercise science in the early twentieth century, physiologists have proposed a number of definitions of low-intensity exercise, which is to say they have proposed a number of different placements for the dividing line between low intensity and moderate. In recent years, however, there has been growing agreement among scientists that this boundary belongs at the first ventilatory threshold because of the abrupt leap in stressfulness that occurs when it is breached.

For runners, the important thing to understand about the VT$_1$ is that it's not really very intense. Research has shown that, for the majority of trained runners, this threshold falls between 77 and 81 percent of their maximum heart rate, between 60 and 65 percent of their maximum aerobic speed (defined as the fastest pace a runner can sustain for about six minutes), and at a rating of 4 on a 1-to-10 scale of perceived effort. To make this more concrete, consider the example of a runner whose best 10K time is forty-five minutes flat. A runner of this ability might have a maximum aerobic speed (MAS) of about 9.4 miles per hour or 6:23 per mile, 65 percent of which is 6.11 miles per hour or 9:49 per mile, making this runner's ventilatory threshold pace a full 2:25 per mile slower than their 10K race pace.

How many forty-five-minute 10K runners do 80 percent of their training at 9:49 per mile or slower? Not many—and that's a problem, as you will soon see.

THE MODERATE-INTENSITY RUT

Research has shown that, whereas nearly all elite runners do about 80 percent of their training at low intensity, very few nonelite runners do the same. A 1993 study by Muriel Gilman of Arizona State University, for example, found that less than half of weekly training time was spent at low intensity in a group of female recreational runners.

More recently, Giovanni Tanda of the University of Genova tracked a group of twenty-two recreational runners during their preparation for a marathon. In a paper published in the *Journal of Human Sport and Exercise*, Tanda reported that the runners ran at an average pace of 7:39 per mile in the training process and completed the marathon with an average time of 3:11 (7:18) per mile. Now, VT_1 pace for a 3:11 marathoner is about 8:58 per mile, or eighty-one seconds per mile slower than the runners averaged in their buildup to race day. Even if we assume the subjects of the study incorporated appropriate amounts of tempo running and speed work in their training program, their average pace in easy runs was still probably no slower than 8:00 per mile, or fifty-eight seconds above the limit of their low-intensity range. In short, these runners, like nonelite runners everywhere, were caught in what I call the *moderate-intensity rut*, doing far less of their training at low intensity than the pros do.

Why? Given that elite runners practice the 80/20 principle universally, and that doing so has made them faster, why are most of the rest of us stuck in the no-man's-land of moderate intensity? I believe there are several reasons. One is that recreational runners aren't under as

71

much pressure to employ the most effective training methods. Because we don't risk losing our very livelihood if we fail to maintain the optimal intensity balance, we allow it to be influenced by other factors, such as the common (but mistaken) notion that a run can't possibly do us any good unless it's at least somewhat uncomfortable.

Another reason elite runners spend a lot more time at low intensity than do nonelite runners is that the low-intensity pace range is much broader for the elites, owing to their high level of fitness. The slowest pace at which runners of all abilities—from beginner to elite—feel they wouldn't be better off walking is around thirteen minutes per mile. But whereas a beginner's VT_1 pace might be 11:30 per mile, giving them a functional low-intensity range of just ninety seconds per mile, a pro runner's VT_1 pace could very well be under 6:30 per mile, allowing them to vary their pace far more (and to run much faster) without straying into moderate intensity.

Another factor is mileage. Any pro who attempted to run one hundred or more miles per week while spending half their total training time at moderate and high intensities would explode into a million tiny shards (mild exaggeration). But a nonelite runner who runs, say, thirty miles per week can spend close to half their time at moderate intensity and not even realize it's costing them.

It most certainly is costing them, though. In one study, thirty club runners with an average 10K time of just under forty minutes were divided into two groups and placed on different training programs for a period of nine weeks. Specifically, one group adhered to an 80/20 intensity balance while the other did half their training at moderate intensity, as most nonelite runners do. Both groups ran a little more than thirty miles per week, and both completed a 10K time trial before the training period began and again afterward. On average, members of the 80/20 group improved their performance by 5 percent, while members of the 50/50 group improved by 3.5 percent. This seemingly trivial percentage difference translated into a thirty-five-second difference on the clock, which I think any runner would gladly take. What's more, when the study's authors isolated the results of the six individuals in the 80/20 group who did the best job of adhering to the prescribed intensity ratio, the performance improvement jumped to 7 percent, equal to an additional twelve seconds off their 10K times.

Other research has yielded similar findings. For example, in 2018, Spanish researchers reported that ultrarunners who maintained an 80/20 balance for twelve weeks registered a 2.4 percent improvement in a time-to-exhaustion test, while runners who spent more time at moderate intensity did not improve. The bottom line is this: if you want to get the maximum benefit from your training, you need to do like the pros and slow down.

PUTTING 80/20 INTO PRACTICE

Good intentions alone aren't enough to make an 80/20 intensity balance stick. Bad habits are hard to break, and the moderate-intensity rut is no exception. To succeed in your effort to balance intensities like the pros, you'll need to take the following three steps:

1. Plan: schedule your training with the 80/20 principle in mind.
2. Measure: determine where the line between low and moderate intensity falls for you.
3. Monitor: keep track of your pace, heart rate, or power output while you run to ensure you're at low intensity when you're supposed to be.

Let's walk through these steps one by one.

1. Plan

The 80/20 principle applies to longer timescales: weekly, monthly, and yearly. It does not apply to a single day. In other words, the idea is not to do 80 percent of *every* run at low intensity. Nor should this principle be applied rigidly on *any* timescale. There is no magic in round numbers. You don't need to do *exactly* 80 percent of your training at low intensity to get optimal results. In fact, for the most part, the pros themselves make no conscious effort to maintain an 80/20

73

intensity balance. Instead, they rely on other factors, including a pattern of alternating "hard days" and "easy days" in their weekly workout structure, to ensure that their intensities are balanced appropriately.

Here are a couple of basic guidelines for planning 80/20 weeks: first, plan by time rather than distance. As I mentioned in chapter 3, the effect of running at any given intensity is determined by how much time you spend at that intensity, not by how much distance you cover (though the two are closely related, of course). Second, count all easy runs and long runs entirely as time at low intensity, and count only the fast parts of faster runs as moderate/high intensity. The exceptions are active recoveries between fast intervals, which can be lumped together with the intervals as time spent at moderate/high intensity. Table 4.1 provides an example of an 80/20 training week.

• TABLE 4.1 •
AN EXAMPLE OF AN 80/20 TRAINING WEEK

MONDAY	TUESDAY	WEDNESDAY	THURSDAY	FRIDAY	SATURDAY	SUNDAY	TOTALS
Rest	Interval Run 15:00 easy 5 x 4:00 at high intensity/ 2:00 easy 15:00 easy	Easy Run 45:00 easy	Easy Run 45:00 easy	Tempo Run 15:00 easy 30:00 at moderate intensity 15:00 easy	Easy Run 45:00 easy	Fast-Finish Run 1:00:00 easy plus 15:00 at moderate intensity	Minutes: 385 Minutes at low intensity: 310 Percentage of time at low intensity: 80.5

2. Measure

How do you know if you're above or below the first ventilatory threshold when you're in the middle of an easy run? The bad news is that the only way to determine your VT_1 exactly is through a laboratory-based treadmill test involving specialized equipment that measures your breathing rate. The good news is that it isn't really your breathing rate you want to know—it's the pace, heart rate, or power associated with the VT_1 because these metrics can be monitored during

74

runs to ensure you're not creeping into the moderate-intensity range unintentionally. And here's more good news: there are some simple ways for you to accurately estimate these values.

▶ Six-Minute Test

The vast majority of professional runners use pace as their primary intensity metric, and with good reason. Pace is objective, simple, and familiar. It's also relevant—races are judged by the clock, so why not train by the clock? For this reason alone, even if you choose to train with a heart rate monitor or power meter, I recommend that you also pay attention to pace.

Determining your VT_1 pace is a fairly straightforward process. I mentioned earlier that, for most runners, VT_1 pace falls between 60 and 65 percent of maximum aerobic speed (MAS), and that MAS equates to the fastest pace a runner can sustain for about six minutes. A six-minute time trial therefore can give an accurate estimate of your VT_1 pace. To do it, find a flat, smooth route that's conducive to running fast, warm up thoroughly, and run as far as you can in six minutes. Convert your average pace for the time trial to speed, multiply this number by 0.65, convert back to pace, and you've got the approximate upper limit of your low-intensity pace range.

As an example, let's say you're pretty darn fit and you cover 1.09 miles in those six minutes, making your average pace for the test an even 5:30 per mile. The speed equivalent of this pace is 10.9 miles per hour. That's your approximate maximum aerobic speed. Multiplying this number by 0.65 yields an estimated VT_1 speed of 7.09 miles per hour, which converts to a pace of 8:27 per mile.

Chances are you've never run a six-minute time trial, which means you might mess up the pacing in your first attempt, either starting too slow and realizing you have a lot of gas left in the tank near the end or (more likely) starting too aggressively and hitting a wall. If this happens, just wait forty-eight hours or so and try again. Although the six-minute time trial is kind of painful, it's short enough that it doesn't take a lot out of a runner and can be repeated fairly frequently.

►Heart Rate

If the six-minute time trial isn't challenging enough for you, try the maximum heart rate (HRmax) test. You may recall that, for most runners, the first ventilatory threshold corresponds to a heart rate of 77 to 81 percent of maximum. Because HRmax varies drastically from person to person, the only way to determine your HRmax accurately is to induce it, and the best way to induce it is to run really hard.

First, strap on a heart rate monitor and jog a mile or two. Then run one mile at a moderate intensity (think a 6 on a 1-to-10 scale of perceived effort) before accelerating gradually over the next quarter mile. Finally, run a quarter mile as fast as you can. The highest heart rate reading you see on your watch before you black out is your HRmax.

I'm joking about the blacking-out part, but be forewarned—it's a torturous protocol. Now, suppose you complete this test and get a result of 185 beats per minute. In this case, your VT_1 heart rate falls between 77 and 81 percent of this number, or between 142 and 150 beats per minute. The fitter you are, the likelier it is that your VT_1 heart rate will be near the top end of this range.

►The Talk Test

A less grueling way to get a good estimate of your VT_1 pace, heart rate, or even power, is the well-known talk test. In these days of gadgets and metrics, this simple instrument, which uses speech to assess exercise intensity, strikes some people as too primitive to have any practical value, yet it does. In 2002, Carl Foster of the University of Wisconsin–Lacrosse reported in the *Journal of Sports Science & Medicine* that the talk test was a highly reliable indicator of the VT_1 (as measured by the standard laboratory method) in a group of fit young men and women that included a mix of athletes and nonathletes. Specifically, the VT_1 corresponded to the highest treadmill speed or cycling power at which subjects were able to recite a forty-nine-syllable statement (the Pledge of Allegiance) comfortably.

To re-create this test for yourself, first pick one or more gadgets you'd like to calibrate through it: a GPS watch, a heart rate monitor, a run power meter, or some combination of the three. Find a smooth, flat route, warm up, and then start a process of increasing your speed in small increments every minute. At every one-minute mark, recite a statement of approximately fifty syllables and see if you are able to do so comfortably while noting your pace, heart rate, or power. If you're not sure whether you are able to speak comfortably, it counts as *uncomfortable*. (Foster's team found that, more often than not, subjects were above the VT_1 when they couldn't state with confidence whether they were able to speak comfortably.) If you *can* still speak comfortably, continue with the process until you can't. Your VT_1 is marked by the highest pace, heart rate, or power at which you "pass" the talk test.

The smaller your speed increases are, the more accurate the calibration will be. Treadmills allow for very small and precise speed increases, but be aware that most treadmills are themselves poorly calibrated. Because this test ends at a fairly low intensity (at the border between low and moderate intensity, to be precise), you can repeat it as often as you like. As you familiarize yourself with the protocol, you will become more confident in its results.

Regardless of which method you use to determine your first ventilatory threshold, you're almost certain to discover that it is somewhat slower than your normal "easy" pace. And a part of you is going to doubt that slowing down your easy runs can possibly do you any good. (Trust me, I hear this from athletes all the time.) Nevertheless, I urge you to give it a chance. Not a day goes by that I don't receive a grateful email or a social media message from a runner who read my book *80/20 Running* or followed one of my 80/20 Endurance online training plans and saw great results after overcoming initial doubts and giving the methods a chance. I very much look forward to receiving *your* positive feedback at some point in the future!

BALANCING MODERATE AND HIGH INTENSITY

Like low intensity, high intensity lacks a single, obvious, universally accepted definition. Various physiological dividing lines between moderate and high intensity have been proposed and debated. Lately, however, scientific opinion has begun to coalesce around the second ventilatory threshold (VT_2), which is a sort of physiological bookend to the first ventilatory threshold in that the breathing rate spikes again when it is exceeded.

For most runners, the VT_2 aligns closely with critical velocity (CV), which is the fastest pace that a runner can sustain with a more-or-less stable internal metabolic state. Runners who undergo testing to determine their critical velocity and are then asked to run to exhaustion at this pace usually last between twenty and thirty minutes. In practical terms, then, high intensity is any running pace that is not sustainable beyond twenty to thirty minutes.

You can derive your VT_2 pace from the same six-minute maximum aerobic speed test you use to determine your VT_1. Most runners hit the second ventilatory threshold between 84 and 87 percent of their MAS. Similarly, you can use the maximum heart rate test I described earlier to estimate your VT_2 heart rate, which in the majority of runners lies between 91 and 93 percent of HRmax.

As Stephen Seiler's research has shown, both moderate- and high-intensity running stress the body significantly more than low-intensity running does. But although high intensity is not significantly more stressful than moderate intensity, it does offer somewhat different fitness benefits. This is important, because if spending too much time at moderate intensity is the biggest mistake nonelite runners make in their training, not spending enough time at high intensity is the second biggest.

There are two reasons nonelite runners tend to do very little training—much less than the pros—at high intensity. One is that spending too much time at moderate intensity, as most nonelite runners do, leaves them without a lot of energy or motivation to run at high intensity. The second is that high-intensity runs can be rather uncomfortable and, although every runner is willing to suffer a bit, most of us seem to prefer the gradual simmer of running to exhaustion at a slow or moderate pace to the acid bath of high intensity. If you want to get the greatest possible benefit from the time you invest in your training, however, you'll probably need to spend more time at high intensity, and if you do, you may even acquire a taste for it.

The question is, how much time? We know that you should do about 20 percent of your running at moderate intensity and high intensity combined, but how should that 20 percent be apportioned between the two?

What do the pros do?

Let's first consider the science. In the wake of the discovery that nonelite endurance athletes get better results when they greatly reduce the amount of moderate-intensity training they do, some exercise scientists became enamored of the idea that moderate-intensity exercise should be avoided at all costs, a few even labeling it "toxic." From this notion the concept of *polarized training* was born. Advocates of polarized training believe that runners and other endurance athletes should do most of their training at low intensity, some at high intensity, and *none whatsoever* at moderate intensity.

I'm no scientist, but this concept immediately struck me as problematic for two reasons. One is that, outside of those who compete in the shortest endurance events (400-meter freestyle swimmers, 1500-meter runners, 2000-meter rowers), very few of the world's most successful athletes polarize their training. The other is that race pace for most runners at most distance falls within the moderate-intensity range, and it defies reason to avoid training in the very intensity range you target in competition.

It came as no surprise to me, therefore, when experimental attempts to validate the polarized training approach fell flat. One such study, conducted by Spanish researchers and published in the *Journal of Sports Science & Medicine* in 2019, involved recreational triathletes training for a half-iron-distance event (a 1.2-mile swim, a 56-mile bike ride, and a 13.1-mile run). For twenty weeks, half of the eighteen subjects did roughly 78 percent of their training at low intensity, 19 percent at moderate intensity, and 3 percent at high intensity ("pyramidal" intensity distribution), while the others adhered to an approximate 85/4/11 breakdown (polarized intensity distribution). Contrary to the expectations of the researchers, the pyramidal group improved

79

more in most physiological measures and performed better in the race itself, leading them to concede, "According to our results, coaches should not discard training time [at moderate intensity] in recreational triathletes [training for] a Half-Ironman race."

Keep in mind, *all* the subjects in this study adhered to the 80/20 rule, more or less, and all of them improved. But those who were asked to avoid moderate intensity exercise didn't improve to the same degree. So much for the notion that moderate intensity is toxic. On the other hand, in certain studies focused on race events much shorter than a half-iron-distance triathlon, the polarized approach has acquitted itself much better. So, where does this leave us?

My advice is to forget about science in this instance. Eventually, the folks in white lab coats will catch up to elite best practices in this area. Until then, it's best just to copy the pros, who, quite reasonably, tend to favor moderate intensity when training for longer events and to favor high intensity when training for shorter events. By comparing the training plans for shorter events against those for longer events in chapters 10–14, you'll get a good sense of how this is done.

FROM INTENSITY TO PACING

Up to this point, we've assumed that there were only three speeds at which a runner can possibly train: slow, moderate, and fast. In fact, these three general intensity ranges are just that—ranges—and it's possible to target a variety of specific paces within each range, which is what the pros do. For example, research has shown that training at or very near VO_2max intensity is a potent stimulus for improved aerobic capacity. In order to maximize your aerobic capacity, you need to include workouts that are designed to allow you to spend time at this specific intensity, and not only that, you must also execute these workouts correctly, which is something that no GPS watch, heart rate monitor, or power meter can do entirely for you. Correct execution of this type of workout requires that you complement such objective metrics with appropriate adjustments to your pace based on subjective measures, particularly your perception of speed and effort.

In fact, these subjective metrics play an important fine-tuning role in relation to intensity during runs of all types, including race-pace workouts designed to cap your preparation for specific race time goals and even easy runs, in which your pace needs to fluctuate from day to day in response to how you're feeling. In short, getting the most out of your training requires that the science of intensity balance be combined with the art of pacing, which just so happens to be the subject of the next chapter.

Coach's Tip

The Importance of Variety

Matt and I don't agree on everything about training—it would be hard to find two coaches who do. That being said, we wouldn't be writing this book together if we didn't agree on the big stuff, and that includes the 80/20 approach to balancing training intensities. I definitely talk the talk and walk the walk when it comes to the philosophy of running easy most of the time. In fact, I think it would surprise you just how easy our easy days actually are at NAZ Elite. We take the word *easy* quite literally. Case in point: even this old, washed-up, former quasi-professional runner can hang with the group on a recovery run—well, half of one, anyway.

Of course, the hard days are a different story. We come to *play*. And we play in a bunch of different training zones, all year long, and often hit several different zones in any given workout. We do a lot of work in what we call the steady-state zone, which for the pros is their marathon effort—the pace at which they could race for two to two and a half hours. We also do a lot of work in the lactate-threshold zone—the pace at which they could race for one hour. We run repeats at 10K pace, and 5K pace, and 3K pace, and mile pace. We even do some all-out sprinting. For us, there is no zone that is necessarily more important than any other, though we may emphasize one or two more than the others as we get close to a race that itself emphasizes those particular zones.

The marathon is a good example. When Matt came to Flagstaff to train like a pro for the 2017 Chicago Marathon, he wasn't only focused on long marathon-specific efforts. Over the course of his time here, he ran 200-meter repeats at mile pace, 300-meter repeats at 5K pace, one-kilometer repeats at 10K pace, mile repeats at lactate-threshold pace, and, of course, long efforts of up to fifteen miles at marathon pace. But that's not all. He also did runs based on effort, like hill repeats and fartleks. Once, he even ran 1500 meters as fast as he could—after having already run 7 x 1K at lactate-threshold effort beforehand.

The point is, the pros do not do the same three or four workouts over and over again on repeat—and neither should you. Variety is the spice of life, as they say, and I like to apply that same principle to training. Check out this workout that we have done a few times: It starts with a three-mile effort at steady-state pace, followed by four minutes of rest. Then we run 4 x 800 meters at lactate-threshold pace with a minute's rest after each rep (two minutes after the last one). Then we run a two-mile tempo segment at slightly slower than lactate-threshold pace followed by three minutes of rest. Then we run 4 x 400 meters at 10K pace with a minute's rest after each rep. And, finally, we run a fast mile—slightly slower than 10K pace. Phew! After writing all that down, I realize how hard it sounds. But hard is fun. Hard equals challenging. And to be challenged is what we want.

The cool thing about this workout is that we didn't steal it from anyone. We didn't read about it on the internet or in a book (no offense to myself or Matt). We just knew what we wanted to accomplish, and we came up with it. Actually, I let our team's 2016 summer intern, Patrick Gildea, design this session, so I call it the "PG." I told him I wanted a high-volume session that hit a bunch of different training zones, but where nothing was all-out. And he nailed it. That's the beauty of this whole training thing. When you've been at it long enough, you realize that it's the overall training principles that need to be adhered to, not a set of ten "must-do" workouts carved into stone.

Creating a plan for a training segment is like putting together a puzzle. But the fun part is that each segment is a new puzzle. You are not just taking apart an already completed puzzle and putting it to-

83

gether again. You are creating all new pieces. Not completely new, of course. As with most puzzles, the pieces look very similar, their slight differences almost imperceptible when strewn across the table. When examined one by one, though, each piece is indeed unique.

And in that uniqueness lies the challenge. A new workout, one an athlete has never done before, poses not only a new physical challenge but also a new mental stimulus. Even the professional athletes I coach are extra pumped when they get to test a workout that's new to our arsenal. I believe this was in part what helped Matt set a personal best at Chicago in 2017—every week he was challenged with something he had never done before. A runner his entire adult life, Matt had done plenty of lactate-threshold workouts, plenty of repeats at 5K and 10K pace, and so forth. But he hadn't done these things in the way we were having him do them. And all this novelty had him excited to come to practice every day, even after three decades as a runner.

If I've sold you on the value of mixing things up—if you're now ready to play Dr. Frankenstein and tweak some of your staple hard workouts (or work with your coach to do so)—then great. Just remember the context in which you exercise your creativity. Remember the 80/20 rule. Remember also that these hard workouts need to represent the optimal volume and intensity for *you*. Maybe the PG, for example, is a bit too much for you. That's totally fine. But you know the point of the workout is to hit a bunch of different training zones in one session without ever going all out. Now you have the tools to come up with your own PG. So have at it and enjoy!

5

PACE LIKE A PRO

S IX WEEKS BEFORE THE 2020 Houston Half Marathon, Japanese elite runner Hitomi Niiya sat down with Tsuyoshi Ugachi, a hired pacer, to discuss strategy for the upcoming race, in which Hitomi hoped to set a new national record for 13.1 miles. Two weeks later, Hitomi did her biggest race-specific workout of the training cycle, a track session consisting of 3 x 5000 meters at her goal pace of 3:09 per kilometer. This was followed after another couple of weeks by a final sharpening session of 3 x 3000 meters at the same pace. Hitomi then flew to Houston, where, less than forty-eight hours before the big event, she ran the second half of the course with Ugachi, covering the closing 3000 meters in 9:24, or just under 3:09 per kilometer. On race day, Hitomi utterly destroyed a women's elite field stacked with top American and East African runners, powering away to win in a record-breaking time of 1:06:32, having averaged—you guessed it—just under 3:09 per kilometer.

As this story illustrates, professional runners take pacing very seriously, and they tend to be exceptionally good at it. They know precisely how fast they can go, and they go precisely that fast when it matters. Such mastery of the art of pacing enables the pros to get more out of their fitness than do most nonelite runners, who tend to be less adept at this crucial skill. Fitness is really nothing more than potential, after all. Pacing functions as the mechanism by which this potential is translated to performance, and as such, it is far more important than many runners recognize. The better a runner is at pacing, the less fitness they waste in races and workouts.

In a book titled *Pacing in Sport and Exercise*, exercise physiologists Andrew Edwards and Remco Polman define pacing as "the goal-directed distribution and management of effort across the duration of an exercise bout." Sprinters don't have to worry about distributing or managing their effort—because fatigue does not play a limiting role in their events, pacing is irrelevant. It's only in longer races, where fatigue does limit performance, that distributing and managing effort becomes a key strategic factor. In other words, pacing is *the thing* that distinguishes a sprint from a distance event.

The shortest running event in track and field is the 60-meter dash. Whether you're a good sprinter or a not-so-good sprinter, to do your best in the 60 meters, you start out running as fast as you possibly can and continue running as fast as you can until you hit the finish line. The same is true of the 100 meters and 200 meters. But somewhere between 400 meters (the longest event recognized as a sprint) and 600 meters (the shortest event regarded as a distance event), things change. No longer is the fastest way to reach the finish line an all-out effort from the first step to the last. Instead, it's a paced effort, where the athlete holds back intentionally, running not as fast as they can but as fast as they feel they can go the whole way. It's not easy to get it just right—to finish a race of 600 meters or longer knowing you couldn't have finished any faster by holding back either less or more at various points—and again, most nonelite runners aren't very good at it.

Pacing isn't important only in races, though. It's equally important in training. As we saw in the preceding chapter, a majority of nonelite runners run a little too fast in their easy runs, a costly training error that is fundamentally an error of pacing. In harder workouts, pacing plays a different but no less critical role. Suppose your training plan calls for you to do a workout comprising 8 x 600 meters at 5K race pace, and you run the first couple of reps too fast. As a result, you fatigue prematurely and are forced to lengthen the recovery jogs after the middle reps just to hit the intended target pace. By the time you get to the final rep, you're so deep in the hole that even an all-out effort isn't enough to keep your splits from inflating even further. This is *not* the workout you were supposed to have done, nor will you derive as much benefit from it as you would have gotten from the prescribed session, and it's all because of poor pacing.

To get the most benefit from your training, you need to understand how to pace each type of run properly, and then you need to actually go out and do it. Likewise, to achieve your best possible performance in races, you need to be good at pacing, and an important function of the training process is to develop pacing skill. In this chapter, I will show you how to pace like a pro in your training, with tips on developing pacing skill and guidelines for pacing different types of runs. First, though, let's lay some context with a closer look at the science of pacing.

THE SCIENCE OF PACING

Humans are not the only creatures that have the ability to pace their physical efforts. Consider the cheetah. Zoologists have observed that cheetahs run significantly farther in hunts that end in a successful kill than in hunts that don't. This suggests cheetahs are able to accurately judge whether they are likely to catch their prey, and when they deem success unlikely, they give up the chase in order to avoid wasting energy. Interestingly, the longest unsuccessful chases are usually carried out by young cheetahs, an indication that they do not yet know their limits as well as the more seasoned hunters do.

What is going on in the mind of a cheetah when it makes the choice to either continue the chase or leave off? Two key factors feed into this decision. One is objective information, such as the speed of the antelope and the distance separating it from the cheetah—math, in other words, though not the kind involving conscious computation. The other factor is the cheetah's subjective sense of what it is capable of—how near to the point of exhaustion it seems to be, how much more strain it feels it can handle.

The pacing decisions of human distance runners work similarly. The difference is that our superior intelligence enables us to pace ourselves in more sophisticated ways. A cheetah could never hunt

87

prey that was too far away for it to see, but an experienced runner like Hitomi Niiya is able to comprehend abstract distances well enough to run the early kilometers of a race at precisely the right speed to ensure she neither runs out of gas before she reaches a finish line many kilometers away, nor gets there with any gas left.

No human is born with this ability. Mastering the art of pacing depends as much on experience for us as it does for cheetahs. If you've ever watched children participate in their first fun run, you know this to be true. Common fun-run distances such as one kilometer and one mile mean nothing to them; knowing only that it's a race, they start off at a full sprint, hit the wall after 200 meters or so, and carry an invisible piano on their back the rest of the way. But they learn from their mistake, and in the next fun run they start out a bit more conservatively, and in the next one after that their pacing is better still.

The same experience-based learning process unfolds in adults, as science has demonstrated. In a 2008 study, researchers at the University of Exeter separated eighteen experienced cyclists into two groups, both of which completed a series of simulated four-kilometer time trials on stationary bikes. But only one group was told the distance of the time trials beforehand, while the other group was told only that all four time trials were equal in distance. Quite sensibly, members of this second group rode cautiously in the first time trial, seeking to conserve energy in case the mystery distance was lengthy. In fact, though, it wasn't very long (four kilometers takes only a few minutes to cover on a bike), so their pacing strategy became increasingly aggressive over the next three repetitions until, in the last one, they performed just as well as the nonblinded group.

Experiments like this one show us not only that pacing is learnable but also that, when it is done well, it is done by *feel*. Other studies have found that supplying inaccurate performance data to athletes, causing them to believe they are going either faster or slower than they really are, has no effect on their performance in time trials—further evidence that the body knows best what it can do.

I believe one of the reasons so many nonelite runners aren't very good at pacing is that they've become too dependent on gadgets to tell them how they're doing and what they're capable of, muzzling their own built-in pacing mechanism. A lot of runners I work with seem to wish there were some device or test or formula or calculator that could tell them exactly how fast to go at every step to get from the start line to the finish line in the least time possible. But these things don't exist, and our current scientific understanding of how pacing works suggests they never will—that the built-in pacing mechanism of an experienced runner who has mastered the art will always make better decisions than even the most sophisticated gadget.

The reason—one reason, anyway—is that psychology, not physiology, determines the limits of running performance. Runners can go no faster than they *feel* they can go. When runners hit the wall during competition, there is (except in cases of exertional heat illness and other rare health catastrophes) nothing wrong with them physiologically—no biological reason whatsoever that they can't continue to run as fast as they were previously. They slow down or stop only because they *feel* they are unable to continue at the same pace.

Personally, I'm glad runners can't offload the responsibility of pacing optimization to science or technology. For one thing, it keeps our sport human. Call us old-school, but Coach Ben and I agree that much of the fun would be drained out of running if the outcome of each workout and race was foreordained, a matter of speeding up, slowing down, or holding steady in reaction to the infallible android voice in your earbuds. The word *performance* is apposite, because no matter how well prepared you are, it's on *you* to execute in the moment. In much the same way that stage actors must not only know their lines but also deliver them convincingly under the lights to win an audience's approval, you as a runner must pace yourself skillfully to get the most out of however much potential you have on a given day.

The other thing I like about the experiential nature of skillful pacing is that it makes running as much a game of the head as it is a game of the body. There's nothing you can do about the amount of physical talent for running you were born with, but pacing is a completely separate talent, one rooted in perceptivity (the ability to interpret your conscious sense of effort) and intelligence (in this case, the implicit mathematics of distributing your effort optimally over the duration of a run). In this way, pacing is a democratizing element of our sport. There is no reason the slowest runner in a given race can't be the best pacer. Indeed, there is no reason *you* can't be the best pacer in a given race. I encourage you, therefore, to regard pacing not as a daunting nuisance but as a competitive opportunity. In committing yourself to becoming good at something most runners aren't good at, you stand to gain an advantage.

To be clear: where pacing is concerned, there's no substitute for experience, which must be earned. You can accelerate your rate of improvement in this subtle art, however, by taking an intentional approach to improving your pacing ability, like the pros. Every run you do should serve as pacing practice at the same time it serves to build fitness. All it requires is that you start each run with an explicit pacing plan, and that you remain mindful of this plan throughout the run. Additionally, you can gamify the pacing element of your runs in ways that will make them more beneficial as both pacing practice and fitness builders.

PACING GAMES

Some runners have an innate gift for pacing, while others do not. In my experience, natural-born pacers tend to pay more attention than other runners do to both the subjective and objective dimensions of pace when they run, heightening their sensitivity to pace. Many of these athletes play little pacing games during training, such as trying to "negative split" workouts (i.e., complete the second half slightly faster than the first). Triathlon legend Dave Scott, for example, used to run and ride the same routes over and over around his home in Davis, California, getting to know them so well that he could predict his race times with uncanny accuracy based on the times he was hitting on those routes.

Although the word *games* carries associations of frivolity, I believe these mental exercises are a big part of what makes the best pacers so masterful at this subtle art. Before the 1989 Ironman World Championship, Dave Scott raised eyebrows by telling the press he expected the winner (meaning himself) to finish in eight hours and ten minutes, or eighteen minutes below his own course record. Sure enough, Dave completed the race in 8:10:13 (closing with a 2:41:03 marathon in eighty-five-degree heat)—the only problem being that he was fifty-eight seconds behind archrival Mark Allen. Whether or not you possess the psychological hardwiring that distinguishes the Dave Scotts of the world from most runners, you too can become a master pacer by incorporating pacing games into your training.

Guess Your Split

Whereas some pacing games require special workout formats, Guess Your Split is a beneficial pacing game you can play in any run, including the easy runs that are the bread and butter of any sensible training plan. All games are built on rules, and like the old schoolyard playground game Kill the Man with the Ball, Guess Your Split is a game whose rules are contained in its very name. The most basic way to play is to set your watch to auto-split mode and then guess your time before checking it when the device signals a completed mile or kilometer. No matter how bad your guesses are initially, I guarantee you'll get better if you perform this exercise consistently.

Other versions of the Guess Your Split game work well in different types of runs, including interval sessions. When I was in high school, my teammates and I often did a workout consisting of 12 x 400 meters at one-mile race pace. The stronger runners among us made a game of taking turns leading a lap, at the completion of which the others tried to guess the split. By the end of the track season, we were so dialed in that any estimate straying more than a few tenths of a second off the mark was judged an epic fail.

Mastering the art of pacing is really all about aligning objective metrics with subjective perceptions. It is, in other words, about gaining a more and more refined sense of what eight minutes and twenty-two seconds per mile (or whatever) feels like, and of what your perceived effort should be when you're, say, four kilometers into a 10K race. The Guess Your Split game is a simple and effective way of pushing this calibration process forward.

91

The Metronome Challenge

Let's return to that 12 x 400 workout that my high school teammates and I did back in the day. Suppose that, instead of taking turns leading laps and guessing split times, we had tried to run each 400 in precisely the same time. That's the Metronome Challenge.

Unlike the Guess Your Split game, which you can apply to any run type, the Metronome Challenge works best in interval workouts featuring multiple repetitions at a uniform distance. There are two versions of the game. The first entails choosing a specific time for each repetition and trying to nail it from start to finish. This version is ideally suited to workouts whose main purpose is to give you practice in running at goal pace for an upcoming event. Maybe you're sharpening up for a 5K road race and your goal is to break twenty minutes. In this scenario, a good workout to do as a final sharpener is 5 x 1K at goal pace, or 4:00 per kilometer. From a physiological perspective, it makes no difference if your splits for the five repetitions are 4:01.2, 3:59.6, 3:59.9, 4:02.0, and 3:58.1 or 4:00.0, 4:00.0, 4:00.0, 4:00.0, and 4:00.0. But striving toward the latter outcome will give you both the desired physical benefit of the session and pacing practice that could prove difference-making on race day.

The second version of the Metronome Challenge is appropriate for workouts where you're targeting an intensity (say, VO_2max) rather than a pace. In this case, instead of choosing a bull's-eye number ahead of time, you might aim to run the first repetition within the appropriate intensity range and then try to complete each subsequent repetition in exactly the same time, assuming it falls within the targeted range.

The Guardrail

In June 2017, just over a week before I left home to join NAZ Elite for the summer, I got my first taste of the Guardrail, a workout invented by Coach Ben. To ensure I arrived in Flagstaff prepared (or as prepared as I could be) for the rigors of pro-style training, Ben started coaching me remotely a few weeks in advance, and the Guardrail was one of several unfamiliar workouts he put on my schedule. The version he gave me consisted of ten uphill intervals wherein my job was to cover slightly more distance in the span of one minute each time. The original Guardrail is a workout of similar design that the NAZ Elite crew tackles every once in a while on a particularly nasty hill in Flagstaff. Although not explicitly intended as pacing practice for them, I've found it serves this purpose quite well for the athletes I coach.

What I like about the Guardrail is how it challenges runners to slice their perception of pace very thinly. You could make it easy on yourself, of course, by cruising the first rep to give yourself plenty of space for nine subsequent speed increases, but if you did this you'd only be cheating yourself. The proper way to do the Guardrail is to run the first rep at the highest speed that leaves you just enough space for nine small speed increases. The last rep should be an all-out effort.

When I did my first Guardrail in June 2017, I carried a pair of brightly colored socks to use as markers. At the end of the first rep I dropped a sock, which I retrieved on the way back down the hill following the second rep, having dropped the other sock. With the aid of this device, which I highly recommend, I succeeded in covering eight to ten additional feet in each and every rep after the first. Five days later, I competed in a 10K road race. Having estimated that I was ready to run thirty-five minutes flat, I finished in 34:59. That's what pacing practice does for you!

Fastest Mile Last Rule

Nearly 80 percent of runners hit the wall in marathons, slowing down significantly in the last several miles. In some cases, the problem is fitness—the runner simply lacks the endurance to cover 26.2 miles at any speed without slowing down. In most cases, however, hitting the wall is a consequence of poor pacing, something the runner could have avoided by slowing down intentionally in the early miles.

Even the pros sometimes crater in marathons and other long races, but it happens most often among runners who also have a tendency to lose speed in their long training runs. In allowing this bad habit to persist, these individuals are essentially training themselves to hit the wall. But the consequences of poor pacing in long runs don't stop there. Any running you do after you've started slowing down involuntarily offers no benefit. Your body can absorb only so much training stimulus in any single run. When you can't help but slow down, your body has absorbed as much stress as it can successfully adapt to on that day. Beyond that point, you're no longer training, you're just punishing yourself.

Yet another consequence of fading in long runs is that it increases both recovery needs and injury risk. Running form tends to break down at high levels of fatigue, and when form breaks down, tissue damage accumulates in the muscles, bones, and connective tissues. Even if this damage doesn't result in plantar fasciitis or runner's knee or some other overuse condition, it will leave you less ready for the next run.

The Fastest Mile Last Rule is a pacing game that teaches runners to distribute their effort more effectively over longer distances. As with Guess Your Split, the name of this particular game is also its one and only rule. To play, all you need to do is make sure the final mile of your long run is faster than any preceding mile. It's absurdly simple, but I have found that this approach yields better results than merely telling runners who struggle with long runs to start slower. There's something about gamifying an intention that manipulates human psychology in a helpful way.

The goal is not to blast your final mile as hard as you can. You're just trying to conserve enough energy to complete this mile a few seconds faster than your fastest preceding mile without undue suffering. It's okay to err on the side of caution and start the run at a pace that turns out to be slower than necessary to ensure you finish strong. Nor is it the end of the world if, on your first attempt, you screw up and fade at the end of the run despite trying to obey the rule. Over time, you will move steadily in the direction of being able to complete your long runs at a fairly steady pace that is neither needlessly conservative nor a setup for a late fade.

If you're a metric runner, the Fastest Kilometer Last Rule, while not as catchy, works just as well.

Billat Accelerations

In her book *The Science of the Marathon and the Art of Variable Race Running*, Véronique Billat, whom I first mentioned in chapter 4, describes a workout of her own creation that teaches pacing skill in a unique way. It consists of long, gradual accelerations that last from three to eleven minutes and go from an easy jog to an all-out sprint. The challenge lies in speeding up continuously without running out of gears before the end point, and it's harder than it sounds, requiring you to focus on your perception of speed and effort far more intensively than you do in any other type of workout.

After testing various formats on the athletes I coach, I've come up with three that I like especially. The introductory version features accelerations of eleven and three minutes, each followed by a lengthy walk-to-jog recovery (trust me, you'll need it); the intermediate level includes accelerations of eleven and six minutes; and the advanced format has all three accelerations (eleven, six, and three minutes). These workouts are incorporated into some of the training plans presented later in the book.

HOW TO PACE YOUR TRAINING RUNS

The Fastest Mile Last Rule is more than just a useful pacing game; it's also a good general guideline for long-run execution. Proper pacing is essential to getting the intended benefit not only from long runs, but from all run types, including easy runs, runs that target a specific intensity, and runs that target a specific pace.

Easy Runs

When I first joined NAZ Elite as an honorary member at the beginning of the summer of 2017, I couldn't keep up with the team's real, full-time members in any type of training run, including easy runs. More accurately, I *could have* kept up, but it wouldn't have been wise, because those runs would no longer have been easy enough for me. By the end of the summer, however, I was able to hang with the real pros in some of my easy runs without pushing too hard. Two things had changed by then. One was that I had gotten fitter. The other was that the pros were going slower in their easy runs, not because they *hadn't* gotten fitter but because they were training much harder than before, and slowing down their easy runs was a necessary adjustment that kept them from becoming so fatigued they couldn't perform well in key workouts.

For me, this experience served as a valuable reminder of the vital role that easy runs play in the training process, and of the importance of taking a flexible, perception-based approach to pacing them. The main function of easy runs is to supply runners with a lot of exposure to low intensity. In chapter 4, we saw that the upper limit of the low-intensity range is the first ventilatory threshold (VT_1) and that most nonelite runners tend to do their easy runs slightly above this threshold. This means most nonelite runners need to slow their easy runs down to maximize their intended benefit. But by how much? Is it enough to slow down to a pace that's just below the VT_1? How slow is too slow?

Here's how I look at it: first off, while in principle it is possible to run too slow in easy runs, I've never actually seen or heard of any runner ever doing it. So don't worry about that. The greater risk—which I *have* seen happen—is trying to do every easy run just below the VT_1 in the belief that doing so will maximize the benefit of low-intensity running. My own view is that the proper way to truly maximize the benefit of your low-intensity runs is to emulate the pros by allowing your pace to vary widely between easy runs, and even within them.

The reason the pros allow their easy pace to vary (while always remaining at low intensity) is that it's the least disruptive way to adjust a training plan in the course of executing it for the sake of ensuring it's neither too heavy nor too light. Before you begin any new training cycle you should, of course, devise (or choose) a training plan. In doing so, however, you need to bear in mind that training plans are fundamentally predictive in nature. They are built upon educated guesses as to how much running is appropriate for you to do, how challenging your key workouts should be, and so forth. But even the best training plan will contain some bad guesses, which means you need to be ready to tweak it as you go.

It's best not to change things unnecessarily, though. Running by feel during easy runs helps you avoid major changes—such as scrapping key workouts due to fatigue—by allowing you to adjust your training load upward (by running faster when you feel fresh) or downward (by running slower when you feel tired) as you go. This approach makes a lot of sense because, whereas no single easy run is terribly important, easy runs collectively account for the bulk of your total training stress, so they offer abundant opportunities to micro-adjust your training on the fly and turn a good plan into a great one.

The way to do this is to try to maintain a consistent comfort level throughout all your easy runs, even if doing so results in your pace being not at all consistent. Ideally, you will feel very comfortable from the beginning to the end of every easy run you do. On days when you're carrying fatigue from recent hard training or you're just feeling flat for no particular reason, staying comfortable may require you to run well below your VT_1 pace. But on days when you're feeling good, you may be comfortable right at VT_1 pace, and there's no reason not to hang out there if you're feeling up for it. And, if you're like me, and you often feel bad and good at different points within a single easy run, you can and should allow your pace to fluctuate.

How you feel during your easy runs is not arbitrary. Use this information about how your body is doing to determine what sort of training stimulus is appropriate. By allowing comfort to set your pace, you will not miss opportunities to run faster and get a bigger training stimulus when your body's up to it, but at the same time you will avoid overtaxing your body when it requires a gentler training stimulus. The long-term effect will be that your overall training load stays within the Goldilocks zone—high enough but not too high.

Workouts with Intensity Targets

In pro-runner parlance, *workouts* are runs containing substantial efforts at moderate or high intensity. Easy runs and low-intensity long runs are *not* workouts in prospeak. Interval runs, tempo runs, and hill repetitions runs are.

Some workouts target a certain physiological intensity, while others target a particular pace (usually a pace associated with a specific race distance, e.g., mile race pace). A slightly different approach to pacing is required by each. In workouts that target a physiological intensity, the goal is to *conform your pacing to the structure of the workout*.

Consider a hill repetitions run comprising 5 x 2:00 "hard" uphill with 3:00 jog-back recoveries. The proper way to execute a session like this is at a 90 percent effort. This does *not* mean you start the first rep at 90 percent of your maximum sprint speed and try to sustain this speed all the way through the end of the last rep—that would destroy you. What it does mean is that you consider the session as a whole and aim to finish it feeling you could have run the reps 10 percent faster, if you'd had to, or you could have run 10 percent farther at the same speed. If you succeed in this aim, you will be able to describe this workout afterward as difficult but not grueling.

Another example is thirty-fifteen intervals, a personal favorite of mine. This workout consists of alternating segments of thirty seconds "on" and fifteen seconds "off," where the "on" segments are taken at a pace the runner could sustain for about fifteen minutes and the "off" segments are active (jogging) recoveries. The introductory version of this session comprises three sets of 8 x 0:30 on/0:15 off with 3:00 of easy jogging between sets. The intermediate version features ten-rep sets and the advanced version twelve-rep sets. Although the target intensity is associated with a specific pace and a specific heart rate for each runner, the "on" segments are so short that neither of these metrics is a particularly useful guide. It's better just to try to manage your effort by again aiming to complete the workout feeling it constituted a 9-out-of-10 effort overall.

If you're like most of the athletes I coach, you'll completely blow the pacing in this session the first time out, starting too fast and then paying the price later. The road to pacing mastery is paved with pacing errors! Understanding what it means to pace workouts of this sort correctly will ensure you get them right eventually.

Not all workouts targeting a specific intensity are intended to be equally challenging. In pro-style training, each week contains two or three key sessions, one or two of which are designed to increase a particular component of fitness while the other one or two function to merely maintain a fitness component and are therefore less challenging. One of Coach Ben's favorite sessions for maintaining leg speed consists of 10 x 20-second relaxed sprints with 1:00 of active recovery between hard efforts. It's tougher than an easy run, certainly, but there are far more taxing speed workout formats out there, and that's the whole idea. This session does just enough to maintain speed when other fitness components are a higher priority.

Where pacing is concerned, it's helpful to understand the *spirit* of each workout—not just the intensity that's targeted but also how difficult it's intended to be. To help you with your pacing, the training plans presented in chapters 10–14 incorporate a coded shading system. Darker shading indicates a workout intended to be highly challenging. Lighter shading means a moderately challenging run. Unshaded boxes, of course, signal the easiest runs.

Workouts with Pace Targets

Workouts that target a specific pace are both the simplest and the most difficult to pace correctly. They're simple in that all you have to do is hit the prescribed pace, yet hard in the sense that such targets are the running equivalent of a bull's-eye on a dartboard. The key thing to keep in mind in approaching this type of workout is that it is the effort to nail the targeted pace that matters, not actual success in the effort (though of course you do want to succeed).

An example of a workout targeting 10K race pace is 6 x 0.75 mile at 10K pace with 0.25 active recoveries between reps. Suppose your goal time for an upcoming 10K race is to squeak under forty minutes, which equates to a pace of 6:26 per mile. Your target time for each 0.75 rep, then, will be 4:04.5. You can be sure that you will get the same physiological benefit from this workout whether you complete all six repetitions in exactly this time (a feat for which you would deserve some kind of award) or not, as long as you do not stray more

99

than a couple of seconds in either direction in any single rep. Also, having made a good-faith effort to pace yourself perfectly will increase the likelihood that your pacing is on point in the race itself.

As with workouts that target an intensity, not all workouts targeting a specific pace are intended to be super challenging. There are moments in the training process when a light dose of running at a given target pace is sufficient. For example, your first taste of half-marathon-pace running in the early part of a training cycle leading up to a half marathon should be fairly light. The shading system I described in the previous section will let you know what sort of challenge to expect from each pace-targeting workout.

The rest is up to you.

Running Fast and Relaxed

In high school, I had an interesting conversation with a lacrosse player that I remember to this day. We were talking about training for the mile when he asked a question that stopped me short: "If you want to run a mile as fast as possible, why don't you run a mile every day as hard as you can and just keep getting better and better?"

I had no good answer to this at the time. All I knew was that our coach had us train very differently from the way my classmate suggested. Instead of having us go all out every day, he divided us up into what he called "work groups" based on our 5000-meter times and the amount of running we had done over the summer. Coach was a stickler for pace—he didn't carry around a laminated pace chart for nothing. If we were doing 400s, we had a very specific pace at which to run them; same for 800s, and miles, and tempo runs.

Never did the pace targets Coach gave us require us to run as fast as we could over a given distance. And if you think about it, it's much the same in races. Yes, the point of a race is to run a particular distance as fast as you can, but you're never really running all out until the very end. We do not sprint until we can sprint no more, and then slow to a run, and then to a jog, and perhaps even have to walk it in. Instead, we parcel out our energy over the course of the entire distance, aiming to do so perfectly so that with only a small percentage of the race left we are able to empty our last bit of energy into one final bit of all-out running.

If we can agree that you're actually only running as hard as you possibly can for a relatively miniscule part of the race, then why on earth would we spend a huge percentage of our training running at that sort of effort? My lacrosse buddy might think it would make race pace "feel" easier, and that theory is reasonable. But in practice, that's just not how it works.

What I understand now is that when you maintain a given pace for a particular workout, assuming that pace is optimal, you begin to conquer the mind's natural defenses against running fast. The brain's number one job is to protect us at all times. When we engage in an activity that, if continued for a long enough period of time, would seriously harm us, unconscious areas of the brain begin to send signals to our conscious minds that we should stop. When running a 400-meter repeat at our 5K race pace, even though that repeat only takes somewhere between one and two minutes for the typical high school cross-country runner, the brain goes into Nostradamus mode and predicts that were we to keep running at this pace, eventually we would get dangerously tired. We might cramp up. We could pass out. So the brain gives us the high sign in the form of physical discomfort and loss of motivation that encourages us to quit long before we are actually in any real danger.

Realizing this fact, and acknowledging it, is a wonderful thing. It gives us the power to override these signals; first in practice, and eventually—hopefully—on race day. One of the best ways to achieve this effect is by doing a lot of very structured workouts where you're forced to lock into a specific pace. In locking into a pace, you're essentially pretending you *can't* slow down, forcing yourself to stick to it regardless of those danger signals. To succeed in this effort, you must learn to relax while still running fast. Come race day, you're able to fall back on all of this practice and do essentially the same thing, running relaxed and fast so you're able to complete the distance at a pace that represents your true limit rather than what your brain tries to tell you is your limit.

Here are some staple workouts that I have used over the years to practice locking into a pace that I believe forces the athlete to run

102

fast and relaxed. All of these sessions have a good bit of volume, which allows you to be challenged over the course of the workout in a variety of ways. Early on, the task is to avoid going too fast and wasting physical energy. As the workout progresses, you must stay very present and not worry about what's to come—saving mental energy. And toward the very end, you must be conscious of keeping your form from breaking down and will be forced to pick up the effort in order to continue hitting a pace that felt so easy not too long ago. Sounds a bit like what goes on in your mind and body during a race, doesn't it?

1. 12–20 x 400 at critical velocity (i.e., thirty-minute race pace) with 200-meter jog recoveries
2. 6–10 x 800 at forty-minute race pace with one-minute rests
3. 8–15 x 1k at lactate-threshold pace (i.e., one-hour race pace) with one-minute rests
4. 3–5 x 2 miles at ninety-minute race pace with 800-meter jog recoveries
5. 2–3 x 3 miles at steady-state pace (i.e., two-hour race pace) with one-mile jog recoveries
6. One-hour and fifteen-minute continuous steady-state run at two-hour and ten-minute race pace

Notice again the variety of different training zones. In my experience, it's the act of repeated running at a certain pace that prepares the athlete for the rigors of race day rather than the pace itself. For example, in the spring of 2019, Stephanie Bruce was preparing for the USATF Half Marathon Championships on May 5. In the final month leading up to the race, she ran some of the very workouts I just listed, including 3 x 3 miles and a long steady state. She was as strong as I had ever seen her, and the work paid off—she won the national title by twenty-one seconds courtesy of a blistering final mile.

The next day, Steph asked me if she could run a 5000-meter race on the track on May 16. Mind you, we had done absolutely nothing that would be considered traditional 5000-meter training. No 400s or 800s at 5000-meter race pace. No superfast 200s. In fact, in the entire month of April, she had only stepped foot on a track twice. But I let her do it. And guess what? On race day, she ran 15:17.76—a personal best by more than twenty-five seconds and a team record (since broken). She found a new limit at the 5K distance because she knew how to find her limit at virtually any distance—because she knew how to run fast and relaxed, and because we do a ton of pacing practice. As she and I often say, and as I hope you've gathered from this tip, "When you're fit, you're fit."

STRIDE LIKE A PRO

NOT ONCE IN THE thirteen weeks I spent with NAZ Elite in 2017 did I see Coach Ben correct a team member's running technique. Nor did he meddle with the way I ran (unless you count his occasional gentle teasing about my goofy arm swing). This wasn't because Ben doesn't know or care as much about technique as other elite-level coaches. Had I joined up with a different professional running team and worked with a different coach, I would have experienced a similar nonemphasis on the technique element of running, and that's because technique simply isn't emphasized in elite running the way it is in other sports such as swimming and baseball.

"Why not?" you ask. Is it that runners who reach the pro level already have their form dialed in, so little or no additional tweaking is required? If this is true, then technique instruction is needed only at lower levels of the sport and its main purpose is to make our strides look more like those of the elites. Or is it because technique instruction just isn't an effective way to improve running performance at *any* level?

Fortunately, science offers a clear answer to the question we've posed. While it's certainly true that good form is part of what makes elite runners elite, research indicates that copying the way the fastest runners run does not make the rest of us faster. This doesn't mean you're stuck with the stride you have, however. Every runner's stride evolves automatically over time, becoming increasingly efficient.

What's more, you can accelerate this natural process by practicing the methods the pros use (beyond merely running) to increase their stride efficiency. But before we discuss these methods, let's first define good running form and understand why it can't be taught.

WHAT IS GOOD RUNNING FORM?

If you ask the average running coach what good running form looks like, the answer will probably include phrases like *midfoot strike, high stride rate*, and *low vertical oscillation*. These and other characteristics are indeed common in top runners and less common in slower runners. But there are plenty of exceptions. Meb Keflezighi won the New York City Marathon and the Boston Marathon as a heel striker. Ryan Hall set an American record of 59:43 in the half marathon with an unusually bouncy stride (or a high degree of vertical oscillation, as the biomechanists would say). Mo Farah won ten Olympic and World Championships at 5000 and 10,000 meters with an exceptionally low stride rate.

Given the fact that elite runners have widely varying running styles, it seems unlikely that biomechanical features such as a high cadence can properly define good running form. Further evidence against the idea that one particular style of running is best for everyone comes from studies in which runners are required to change their form to make it more "textbook." Such studies have shown repeatedly that when runners attempt to consciously alter their natural stride in *any* way, they get worse at running, not better. For example, a 2005 study led by George Dallam of Colorado State University Pueblo found that twelve weeks of supervised training in the POSE Method, which emphasizes a forefoot strike, left a group of eight experienced triathletes with significantly reduced running economy.

In all likelihood, it wasn't the switch from heel striking to forefoot striking itself that made these athletes less efficient. Rather, it was the increased mental effort that altering their natural form required of them. Believe it or not, simply *thinking* about one's body movements while running reduces running economy, even when no attempt is made to run differently. Proof of this comes from a series of studies led by Linda Schücker of the University of Münster, who has found that runners move less efficiently when asked to think about their movements while running than when asked to focus their attention externally.

The reason that thinking about running while running makes a runner's stride less efficient is that *self-consciousness* is the enemy of efficiency. This is true not only in running but also in all motor skills. Basketball players shoot free throws less accurately when thinking about their release than when focusing on the back of the rim. Weight lifters deadlift less weight when thinking about contracting their muscles than when thinking about driving away from the floor. Even swimmers move less efficiently when concentrating on *pulling their hand* back through the water than when concentrating on *pushing the water* back with their hand.

Mastering any motor skill is all about automation. The more unconsciously you are able to do anything—from throwing darts to driving a race car—the more skillfully you will do it. Brain activity is proven to steadily decrease as beginners gain experience in a particular motor skill. In a 2017 paper published in *Sport, Exercise, and Performance Psychology*, for example, British researchers showed that neural activity in brain areas associated with conscious processing decreased while performance improved in novice golfers who went through a sequence of three putting practice sessions.

If you happen to be a golfer yourself, you know that you'll never advance beyond duffer status if you don't get some technique instruction. The difference between golf and running is that, unlike swinging a golf club, running is a simple and natural movement that most of us learned how to do *without instruction* as toddlers. There is no running equivalent of arcing your backswing behind the midline to put topspin on a chip shot—something very few golfers would ever figure out how to do without coaching. Whereas golfers seek to automate such learned techniques so that they can execute them almost unconsciously, runners seek (or should seek) to run with a "quiet brain" because the less active the brain is, the easier running at any given pace feels, and the longer that pace can be sustained. And runners don't need help to learn how to run with a quiet brain.

In a 2012 study, Sharon Dixon of the University of Exeter in England measured changes in running economy in a group of new runners. For ten weeks, these runners trained on their own without any technique instruction. Despite making no conscious effort to improve their form, they achieved an average improvement of 8.4 percent in running economy during this relatively brief span of time. Dixon's team was able to link the improvement to subtle changes in the runners' biomechanics that could never be taught in the way that golfers can be taught how to put topspin on a chip shot.

How, then, did these novice runners discover such biomechanical shortcuts? According to experts in motor learning, when a person performs a skill repeatedly, the brain and the musculoskeletal system are in constant communication, with the brain sending instructions to the body based on a stored "blueprint" for the skill being performed and the body sending proprioceptive feedback to the brain about what and how it's doing. No two repetitions of any skill, including the running stride, are exactly the same. Tiny variations in the stride pattern are monitored by the brain in search of specific, accidental variations that happen to require ever-so-slightly less brain effort and are hence associated with an ever-so-slightly lower perceived effort level. The brain seizes on these discoveries and incorporates them into its blueprint for running. One discovery of this sort doesn't make much of a difference, but millions of running strides may yield thousands of little eureka moments that add up to a far more efficient and effortless stride.

The single most effective way to become a more skillful runner, therefore, is just to run. By doing nothing more than putting one foot in front of the other, over and over, you will move closer and closer to achieving your optimal stride. There is no way to anticipate what this stride will look like, and I can guarantee it won't look exactly like any other runner's optimal stride. In fact, what your stride looks like doesn't really matter, and in this sense the term *running form* isn't even appropriate. It's not good *form* you're truly after but running *skill*, which comes from gradually discovering through unconscious experimentation how to run with a quiet brain.

In a 2020 study published in the *European Journal of Sport Science*, a team of researchers led by Robbie Cochrum of Middle Tennessee State University filmed five runners as they ran and asked 121 coaches to rank them in order of perceived efficiency based on their form. Only 6 percent of these coaches were able to rank even three of the five runners in the correct order of their actual, tested running economy, which is the rate at which a runner consumes oxygen at a given speed and is roughly equivalent to motor vehicle fuel efficiency. Clearly, you can't judge the "book" of running skill by the "cover" of running form!

In fact, I would go a step further and argue that running economy is not even the best measure of running skill. It has long been noted that, although individual runners tend to become more economical with experience, the best runners are not always the most economical, and at any given level of performance—all the way to the top—a high degree of variation in economy is seen. I believe this is because the human organism is not even trying to optimize the energy cost of running. Rather, it is trying to optimize the mental effort required to run, which is consciously perceived in the form of how difficult it feels to run at a given pace. Evidence of this comes from studies showing that in certain instances, such as the transition from walking to running, movement patterns that feel easier are actually less efficient, yet people go with what feels easier. For the most part, perceived effort and running economy move in the same direction. But I look forward to the day when less attention is paid to the energy cost of running at a given speed and more to what I believe is the true measure of running skill: mental effort, which can be quantified both objectively as brain activity during running, and subjectively as consciously perceived effort.

Putting one foot in front of the other may be the most effective way to increase running skill thus defined, but it's not the only way. As I suggested earlier, although pro runners do not take technique instruction from coaches the way, say, baseball players adjust their swing in response to input from batting coaches, they do work to improve their form in other ways. These methods are beneficial for runners at all levels of the sport, and they are the focus of the remainder of this chapter.

Form Drills

What can I say? Tradition is powerful. I have just explained that form, per se, is irrelevant to running performance, and now here I am recommending form drills as a means to become a better runner. Despite their name, though, form drills are not intended to make your stride *look* a certain way. Instead, they work by isolating and amplifying particular components of the stride in order to accelerate the process by which the brain refines its running blueprint through two-way communication with the body.

To this point, exercise scientists have shown little interest in studying the long-term effects of regularly practicing form drills. But the acute effects of form drills have been studied, and it's been shown that, when included in a warm-up, they improve performance in the workout or race that immediately follows. Also, as Coach Ben pointed out to me when he put me through my first drill session with NAZ Elite, every runner who practices form drills consistently gets a lot better at them, so they clearly do *something*.

Pro runners typically do drills as part of their warm-up before every workout and race, and many pros—including those on NAZ Elite—also do a longer drill session following an easy run once or twice a week. There are many good form drills to choose from, but these six will get you started. You can find video demonstrations of them on the 80/20 Endurance YouTube channel.

▶ *Carioca*

Named after the Brazilian dance it resembles, this drill entails running forward while rotating the hips from side to side. You can get a feel for it by jogging in place and rotating your hips first to the right and then to the left, taking four steps per rotation and keeping your upper body facing forward. Complete six rotations, pause, and do the same thing again, but this time rotate first to the left and then to the right. When you're ready to carioca for real, start jogging forward and repeat the same sequence I just described, only stop after you've completed the right-to-left rotations and jog back the other way for the

110

left-to-right rotations. Holding your arms away from your body as you go will help you maintain your balance and coordination.

The key difference between the real, moving version of carioca and the static, practice version is the cross-step. As your hips are coming back toward neutral from the right, cross the right leg in front of the left and touch the right foot to the ground ahead of the left (which is now off the ground). Execute a mirror image of these movements when performing left-to-right rotations.

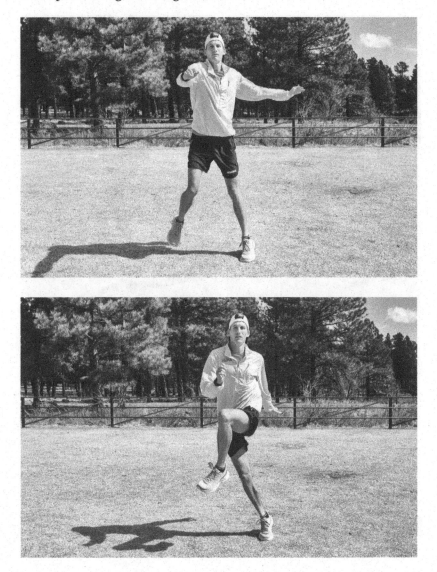

111

▶ *A Skips*

Now for something a little easier: A skips. Lift your right knee high, hop forward on your left foot, and then drive your right foot back to the ground. As your right foot comes down, lift your left knee high, hop forward on the right foot, and then drive your left foot back to the ground. Move your arms just as you would when running while completing twenty skips (ten on each side).

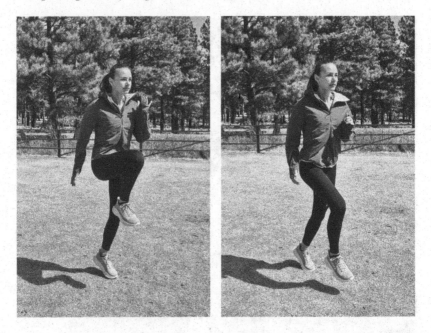

▶ B Skips

B skips are simply A skips with a twist, which is that you snap your active leg to full extension in the process of driving the foot back to the ground, as though you're trying to kick an object out in front of you without interrupting your skipping. Complete twenty skips (ten on each side).

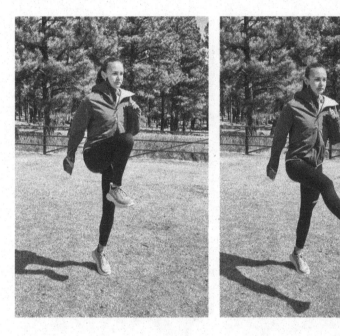

113

▶ *High Knees*

Jog forward while lifting your knees as high as you can at a quick tempo, bringing each foot down directly underneath your hips without letting the heel touch the ground. Keep your torso erect and perform a normal running action with your arms. Complete twenty steps (ten with each leg).

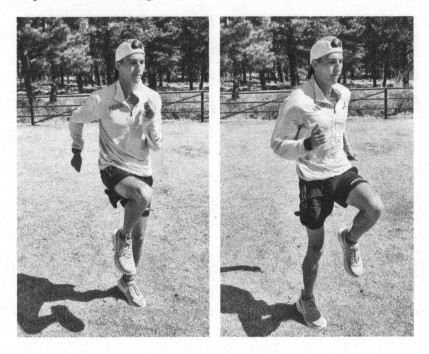

▶ Butt Kicks

Jog forward while trying to kick yourself in the rear end with your heels. Allow your knees to come forward and think about tucking your foot under your saddle area rather than locking your thighs and kicking behind you with your lower legs, which puts a lot of strain on the knees. Take quick steps, stay on the balls of your feet, keep your spine erect, and move your arms as you normally do when running. Complete twenty steps (ten with each leg).

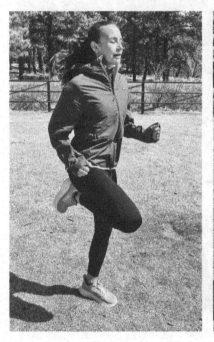 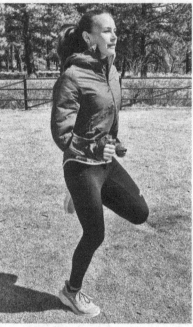

▶ Straight-Leg Running

Jog forward with your knees locked in a slight bend, leaning back slightly and kicking your legs out ahead of your body. Stay up on your toes and perform a normal running action with your arms. Complete twenty steps (ten with each leg).

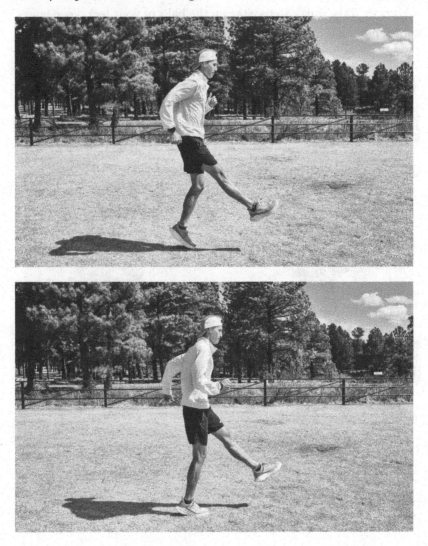

Plyometrics

Roughly half the energy required to maintain a given speed of running is *free energy*, or energy that comes from the ground, not the muscles. When the foot lands, force enters the ground from the body. Some of this force is absorbed by the ground, but the rest rebounds back into the runner's body, creating a propulsive effect. The legs, in other words, function as springs during running. But some springs are more efficient than others.

If you happen to have retained some of the physics you learned in high school, you may remember that springs have varying degrees of stiffness, and that stiffer springs are generally more efficient, able to capture and reuse more free energy than springs that are less stiff. A runner's legs are no exception. A springy runner is able to stiffen their legs on impact and thereby stabilize the joints, minimizing the energy lost through wobbling at the ankle, knee, hip, and pelvis. The results are less ground contact time and better running economy.

Plyometrics, or jumping exercises, are proven to increase leg stiffness and running economy, reduce ground contact time, and improve running performance. A 1999 study by Leena Paavolainen and colleagues at the University of Jyväskylä, for example, reported significant improvements in running economy and 5K race times after nine weeks of plyometric training, as well as a significant reduction in ground contact time.

A little plyometric training goes a long way. Runners who participated in a 2017 study by Chilean researchers experienced significant benefits after six weeks of doing plyos twice per week for less than thirty minutes per session. If you're currently doing little or no plyometric training, you will probably gain something from any amount that you incorporate into your routine. I myself find it most efficient to include plyos in my strength workouts, but you can also combine them with drills during your pre-workout warm-ups or take a cue from NAZ Elite and do a combined session of drills, strides, and plyos after an easy run once a week or so.

Following are four of my favorite plyometric exercises for runners.

117

You can find video demonstrations of these exercises on the 80/20 Endurance YouTube channel.

▶ Single-Leg Drop Jump

On a box that's twelve to eighteen inches in height, stand on your right foot with your left knee bent. Take a gentle leap forward off the box and land on the ground as lightly as possible, stiffening your leg with the knee bent approximately thirty degrees and holding this pose for one second. Return to the box and complete nine more jumps, then do ten jumps on the left foot.

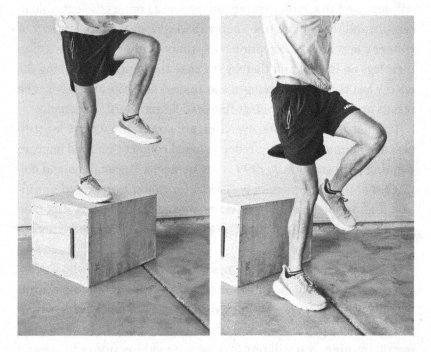

▶ Single-Leg Box Jump

Stand on your right foot facing a twelve- to eighteen-inch box with your left knee slightly bent. Squat down slightly as you naturally do when jumping for height and leap onto the box, landing on your right foot. You may find it helpful to swing your arms back and then forward while initiating the jump to create momentum. Now jump backward down to the floor, again landing on your right foot. Complete nine more jumps and then do ten jumps on your left foot.

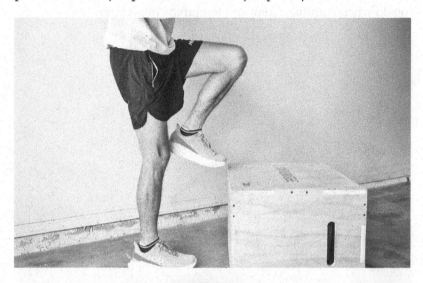

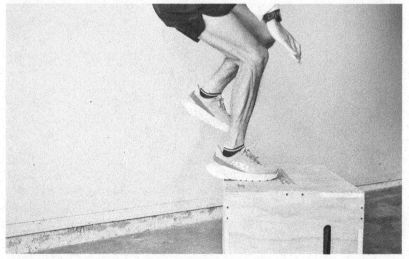

▶ Lunge Jump

Start in a lunge stance with your right foot flat on the ground, your left leg slightly bent, and only the forefoot of your left foot touching the ground, a full step behind the right. Sink down into a deeper lunge, stopping when your right thigh is parallel to the floor, and then leap upward as high as possible. In midair, reverse the position of your legs. When you land, sink down immediately into another lunge and then leap again. Use your arms for counterbalance the same way you do when running. Complete ten jumps in each position.

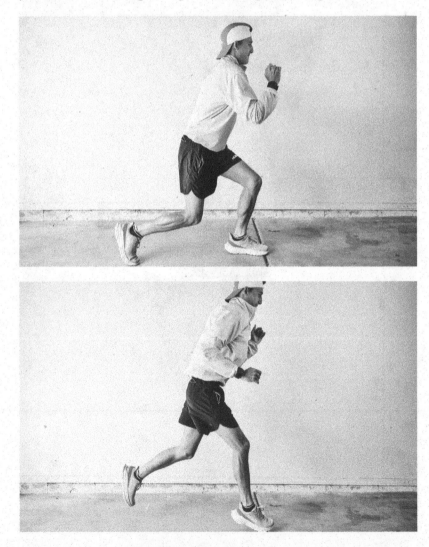

MATT FITZGERALD AND BEN ROSARIO

▶ Toe Taps

Stand facing a box or aerobics step that's eight to twelve inches in height. Start running in place in a modified manner, kicking your legs out in front of your body alternately and tapping the top of the box with the ball of each foot before returning it to the ground directly underneath your hips. Maintain a rhythm that's quick but not hurried, moving your arms in opposition to your legs as you do when running. Continue for thirty seconds.

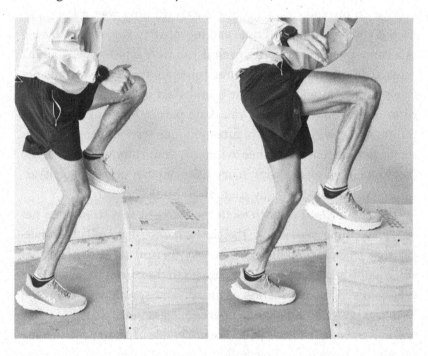

Strength Training

Running skillfully may be all about running with a quiet brain, but that doesn't mean the body is irrelevant. To the contrary, your body can contribute significantly to skillful running by making your brain's job easier. Strength training does this by making the muscles more responsive to the brain's signals and more coordinated in their contractions, and also by delaying muscle fatigue and its negative effect on running economy.

As with plyometrics, a little strength training goes a long way. Even if you had unlimited time and incentive to work on improving as a runner—in other words, even if you were a pro—you wouldn't want to do more than two to three full-body strength workouts per week, as anything beyond that would start to interfere with your running. If you're busy and you don't particularly enjoy strength training, start with a couple of fifteen-minute sessions per week. This small commitment will suffice to improve your running performance (not to mention reduce your injury risk—another proven benefit) assuming you're not doing any strength training currently.

As a runner, you want to focus on exercises that strengthen not only your prime movers (i.e., the glutes, hamstrings, and other muscles that generate propulsive force when you run) but also the smaller and equally important stabilizer muscles in the core, hips, and ankles that help your body function as an efficient spring when you run. Exercises involving balance, independent leg actions, weight-bearing, and movement at multiple joints are preferable because they simulate running in these ways. Bodybuilding-type exercises that add useless bulk to the upper body (e.g., bench press) and machine exercises that develop strength in ways that have little or no functional carryover to running (e.g., machine leg curls) should be avoided.

There are scores of different strength exercises that meet the needs of runners, and I recommend you cycle through a bunch of them in your strength-training routine, as this will eliminate more of your body's weak links than would a more limited and repetitive program. In this spirit, consider the following example of a strength workout just that—an example—and not a perfect or ideal session that you should never deviate from. To do it, you'll need a resistance band, dumbbells, and a stability ball. The eleven exercises that make up the circuit should be completed once each before you go back and do any additional sets. Start with just one full circuit, repeat the workout twice a week, and after two or three weeks add a second circuit if you wish. Adding a third circuit eventually will provide some additional benefit, but I'll leave it to you to decide whether it's worth the extra twenty-minute time investment.

▶ Monster Walk

Loop a high-tension resistance band around your thighs just above the knees and stand with your feet at shoulder width and your knees slightly bent. Take a moderately large step to the right with your right foot. Now take an equal-size step to the right with your left foot, resisting the band's efforts to make the movement quick and jerky. Make sure you keep your hips and shoulders level, and don't deviate forward or backward as you step. Complete ten steps to the right and then ten more to the left.

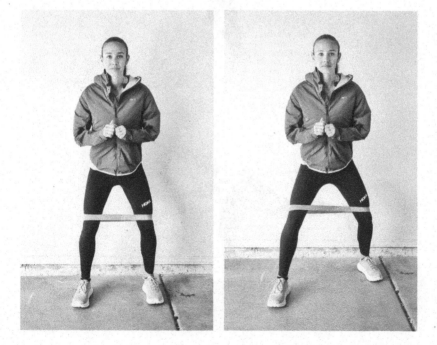

▶ Single-Leg Reverse Deadlift

Stand on your right leg with a slight bend in the knee. Without bending the knee farther, hinge forward at your hip, reaching ahead with both arms and kicking the left leg straight back. Focus on tilting your pelvis until you feel tension in your hamstring and hip. Maintain a normal arch in your back and keep the midline of your torso from swaying to either side. Your pelvis should be level to the floor, the foot and knee of your support leg stable. Pause briefly at the limit of this movement and then return to the start position. Complete ten repetitions and then switch legs.

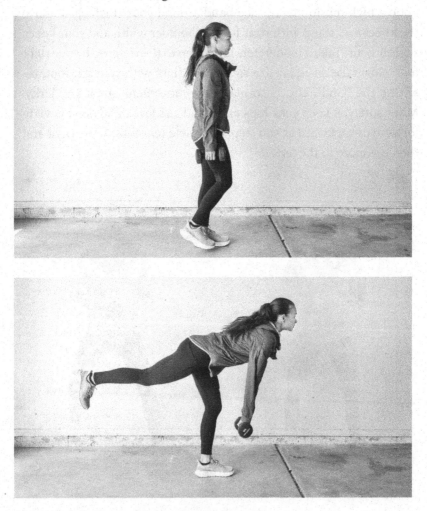

124

▶ Side Plank

Lie on your right side with your left foot positioned just in front of the right one on the floor and your torso propped up by your right arm, which is bent ninety degrees with the forearm resting on the floor. Lift your hips until your body forms a diagonal plank. Hold this position for sixty seconds or ten seconds short of your limit (whichever comes first), making sure you don't allow your hips to sag toward the floor. Switch to the left side and repeat the exercise.

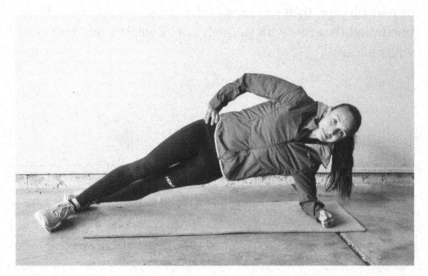

125

▶ Plank Row

Assume a front plank position with your feet together, your body forming a perfectly straight line from heels to shoulders, and each hand gripping the handle of a dumbbell positioned on the floor directly underneath your shoulders. Begin with your elbows locked and your core tight. Now pull the dumbbell in your right hand toward your body in a rowing motion, keeping the rest of your body completely motionless. Continue until the dumbbell touches the outside of your rib cage, then return smoothly to the start position. Pause briefly and then row with your left arm. Complete ten repetitions with each arm.

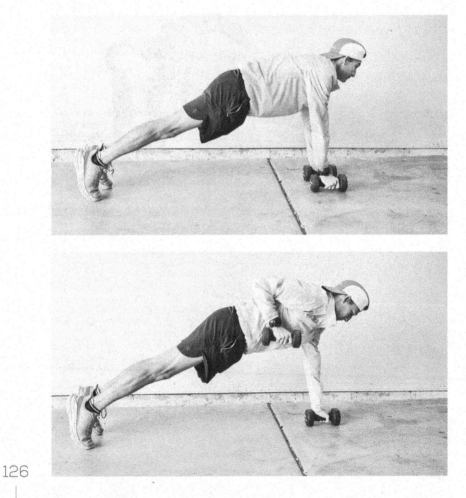

MATT FITZGERALD AND BEN ROSARIO

▶ Reverse Lunge

Stand normally with your arms hanging at your sides and a dumbbell in each hand. Take a large step backward with your left foot and bend your right knee until the thigh is parallel to the floor. Keep your trunk upright and your weight on your right foot. Now press your right heel into the floor and return to the start position. Repeat this sequence with the other leg, and continue alternating until you've completed ten repetitions with each leg.

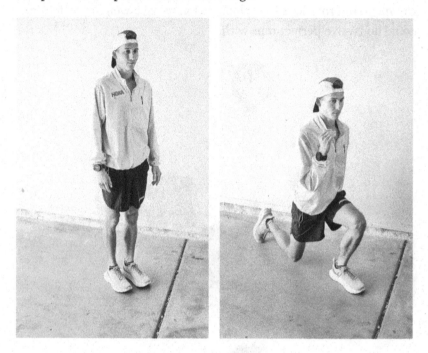

▶ Stability Ball Rotation

Lie faceup on a stability ball with your feet spread wide on the floor, your upper back supported, and your arms extended straight overhead with a medicine ball, dumbbell, or other weight pressed between your palms. Keeping your arms extended, rotate your upper torso to the right and swing the ball toward the wall on that side of the room. Go as far as you can without discomfort or loss of balance and then return to the start position. Now rotate to the opposite side. Complete ten rotations in each direction using a weight you feel you could do twelve perfect reps with.

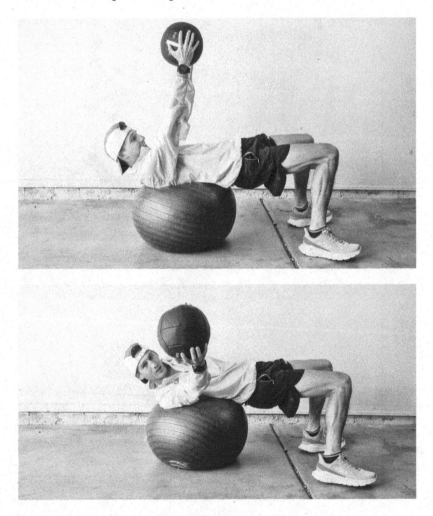

MATT FITZGERALD AND BEN ROSARIO

▶Stability Ball Push-Up

Assume a modified push-up position with your feet together, your body forming a perfectly straight line, and your palms positioned slightly more than shoulder-width apart on a stability ball. Bend your elbows and smoothly lower your chest to within an inch of the ball. Immediately press back upward to the start position. Complete twelve repetitions or two fewer than your maximum (whichever comes first). If you have difficulty doing a full push-up, do a half push-up, bending your elbows only to ninety degrees before pressing upward.

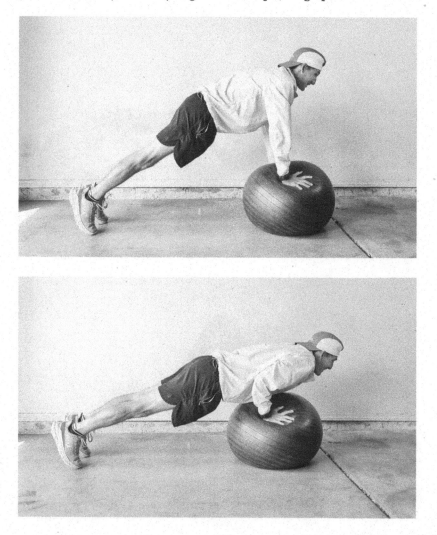

129

▶ *Stability Ball Hamstring Curl*

Start in a bridge position, faceup with your head and shoulders on the floor and your heels resting on top of a stability ball, your body suspended in a straight line between these points. Contract your hamstrings and roll the ball toward your rear end. Pause briefly and extend your legs, rolling the ball back to the starting point. Avoid letting your hips drop. Complete ten to fifteen repetitions. If this exercise is too easy, do a single-leg version, elevating one foot above the ball and pulling the ball toward your butt with the other leg.

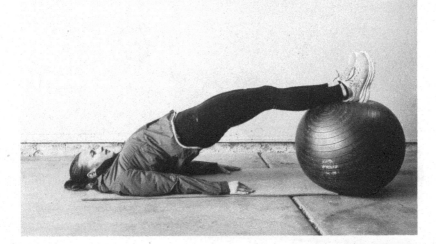

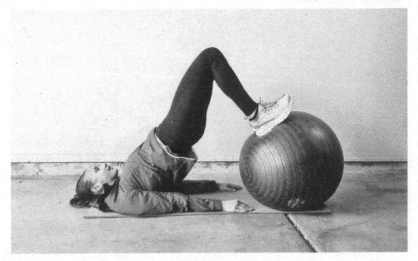

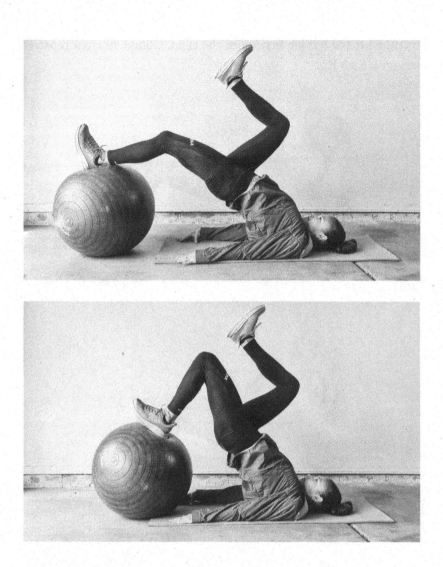

▶ Stability Ball Crunch and Leg Lift

Lie with your back supported by a stability ball and your feet on the floor, spaced at shoulder width, knees bent to ninety degrees. Cross your arms over your chest and rest a palm on each shoulder. Now contract your abdominal muscles and curl your shoulders up off the ball. Holding this position, lift your right foot off the floor and draw the right knee toward your chest as far as you can without losing balance. Lower your foot back to the floor and then relax your abdominal muscles and lie back on the ball. Repeat this sequence, but

131

this time lift the left leg instead of the right. Complete eight repetitions with each leg.

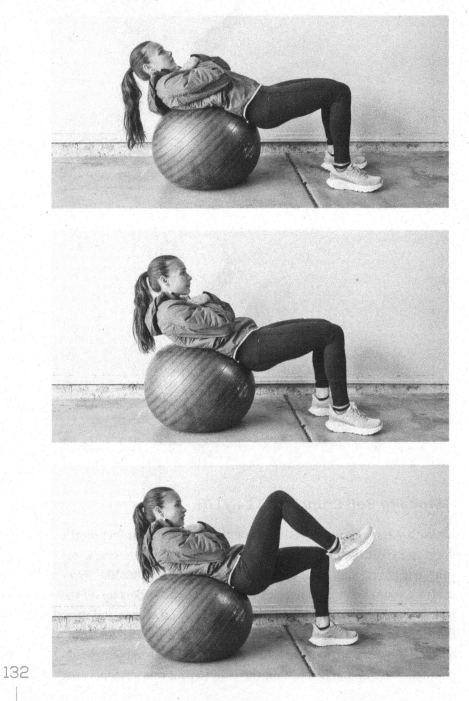

▶ *Wall Angel*

Stand against a wall with your elbows bent to ninety degrees and in line with your shoulders. Eliminate any space between your low back and the wall by tucking your tailbone under your hips. Keeping your elbows, wrists, and shoulders in contact with the wall, raise your arms up above your head as high as possible. Slowly return to the start position and then complete seven more reps for a total of eight.

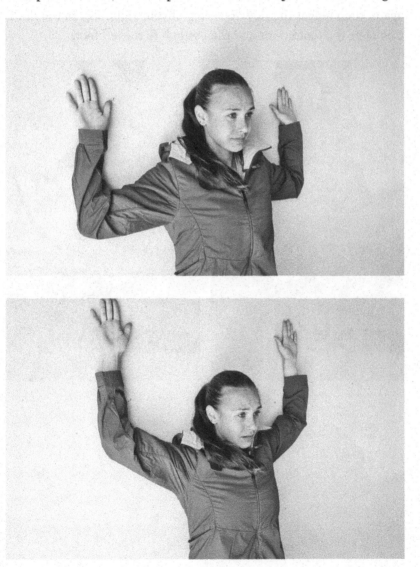

133

▶ Eccentric Heel Raise

Stand normally and contract both calves, raising your heels as high as you can. Now lift your left foot off the floor by bending your knee slightly so that you are supported by the toe of your right foot. (Place a hand on a wall or other stable structure for balance.) Now lower your right heel slowly to the floor on a six-count. When your right foot is flat on the floor, place the left foot next to it and raise your heels again, then repeat the slow lowering of your right heel to the floor. Complete ten repetitions and then switch to the left foot.

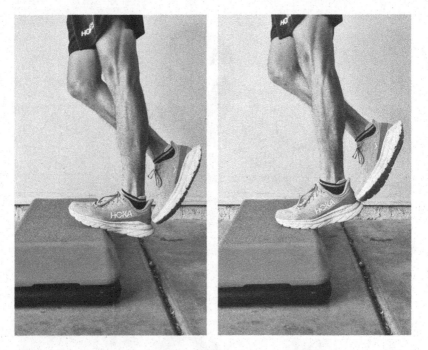

Finding Your Form

Even the best runners have imperfect form. Ethiopia's Haile Gebrselassie, who some consider the best distance runner ever, is a great example. Throughout his legendary career, Geb had a unique, uneven arm carriage; his right arm would swing back and forth while his left arm remained somewhat static. He claimed the quirk was the result of running ten kilometers to school every day carrying his books with his left arm. In any case, the quirk didn't seem to slow him down. The man won ten Olympic and world championship gold medals and set twenty-seven world records for Pete's sake!

My take on running form has long been that it's not about trying to change your form to fit some one-size-fits-all image of perfect technique. It's about figuring out how to take your unique form, quirks and all, and ensure that you're running as efficiently as possible. The goal is to make slight improvements to your personal running style— no more, no less. I've seen plenty of proof that such improvements are possible—and experienced them for myself.

In a previous tip, I mentioned that I ran a 4:03 mile at the age of twenty-nine after spending most of the preceding six years as a marathoner. In that context, I gave much of the credit for this breakthrough to changes in my training mileage and my workouts. But there was another piece to the puzzle, which was that, for the first time since I was in high school, I incorporated plyometric work and a legitimate set of form drills into my training. While my high school coach had been a taskmaster when it came to form drills, my college and professional coaches were not. At twenty-eight years old, I began working with Tim Bradley, who was then the distance coach at

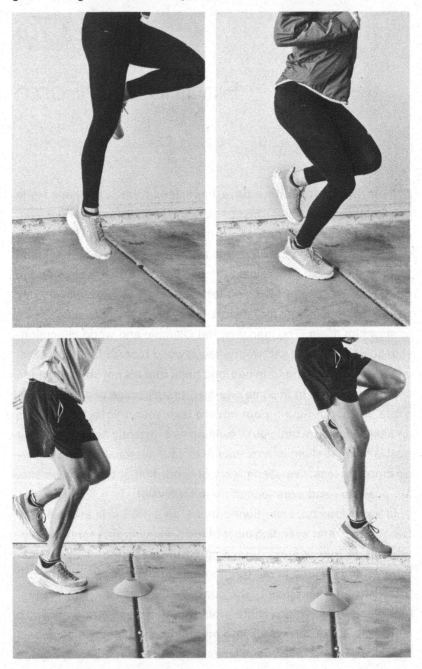

Saint Louis University, on a routine that we hoped would put some spring back in my legs. He had me doing many of the drills that Matt mentioned in the preceding chapter, including A skips, high knees, butt kicks, and carioca.

Tim also introduced me to true plyometric work for the first time in my life. We did single-leg jumps, where the goal was to land on the midfoot and pop right back up off the ground quickly, landing on the same spot each time—five total on each leg. We also did what I called

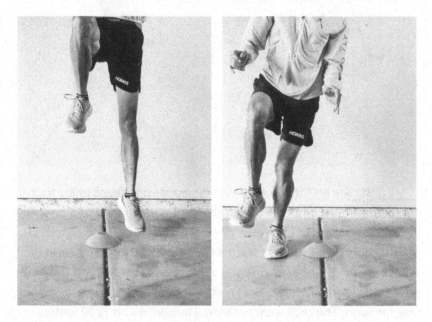

single-leg over-and-backs, standing on one foot and jumping forward over a lane line on the track and back over the same line—again, five total on each leg. A second version of over-and-backs involved jumping laterally over a lane line and then back to the other side.

After I got good enough at these exercises, Tim added cones to the over-and-backs, which forced me to spring higher off the ground with each jump. Finally, we did what he called the fast-feet drill, where I would get up and down off the ground as quickly as possible over a short distance—10 meters or so. It was fun to see the progress I made with the drills and plyos over several weeks; it was translating very tangibly to my running, which was the whole point.

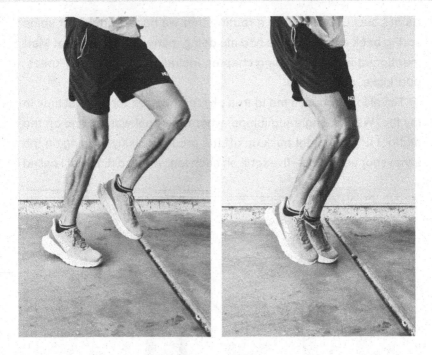

My first race on the track after adding drills and plyos to my training routine was a one-mile indoor race at the University of Missouri.
It was the first meet of the year, in early January, so I didn't expect it
to be terribly fast. But there were a couple of pretty good guys in the
field, including Tipper O'Brien, a 4:02 miler from Mizzou (he had
gone to the same high school I had, so bragging rights were on the
line, for sure). The race went out slow. I believe we hit 1200 meters in
3:13, and then something crazy happened—I just took off, sprinting
like I didn't even know I could. I ran the last 400 meters in fifty-nine
seconds and won the race going away in 4:12. The overall time wasn't
anything special, but the ease with which I had closed the race surprised the heck out of me. To be very honest, it was more fun than it
was hard.

Three weeks later, I had a similar race in Boston, only this time I
came across 1200 meters in 3:06 and ran the final 400 meters in
sixty seconds to finish in 4:06, a time I had never thought possible
for myself. That summer I ran a 4:01 downhill mile on the road and
then it was the next year that I ran my 4:03, also in Boston. Times

aside, I had so much fun in those couple of years, and I can say unequivocally that I would not have run as fast as I did without adding form drills and plyometrics to my training regimen.

Drills and plyos now have an important place in the training we do with NAZ Elite. Our runners have developed a reputation for getting faster with age, and I think these methods have a lot to do with it. As Matt mentioned, nothing improves running economy like running, but in order to keep running consistently year after year you need to support your running with ancillary work, including drills, plyos—and also strength training.

Our runners are fortunate to do their strength training under the expert supervision of brothers AJ and Wes Gregg. Matt just described many of the exercises that are staples in the gym workouts AJ and Wes design for us. More important than any single exercise, though, is the individualized, progressive strength program that they prescribe for each athlete. Steph Bruce and Kellyn Taylor, the two athletes most responsible for our reputation of getting better with age, have been working with the Greggs since 2014. They've done all sorts of exercises, some related to their unique biomechanical needs, some specific to a particular race they're training for, and some intended to address an injury they might be dealing with. Hence, their routine changes from season to season based on any number of variables.

Now, unfortunately we cannot all work with AJ and Wes, two of the best in the business. But you can find professionals in your own neck of the woods. If it's economically feasible for you, you will not regret the investment. Luckily, it's not a case of either/or. Everything we do contributes. Your running technique is uniquely yours, and always will be. It can get better, but that improvement takes time and comes from a variety of areas—none of which should be taken for granted, and all of which require an acknowledgment that perfection is not the goal; it is movement toward perfection that we pursue.

RECOVER LIKE A PRO

A NUMBER OF YEARS ago, I got the opportunity to test a machine that was purported to boost muscle recovery by shooting electrical currents into the muscles. It was loaned to me by an acquaintance who worked as a sales rep for the manufacturer and told a plausible story about how and why it worked. My first impression of the machine was that, if nothing else, it was pretty cool. I definitely felt *something* while I sat on my sofa watching television with several electrodes zapping my legs.

The real test came the following morning, when I did my next run. Would my legs feel any different for having undergone that first treatment? They did not. Nevertheless, I withheld judgment, understanding that not feeling a benefit didn't necessarily mean there wasn't one, and that only with habitual use would any real benefits fully manifest. By the time I returned the machine to the sales rep, however, I had stopped using it. The treatments were kind of inconvenient, and in my gut, I just didn't believe they were worth the bother.

I was far from surprised, therefore, when, years later, researchers concluded that the various types of electrostimulation machines marketed to athletes are a waste of money. A comprehensive review of recovery methods published in *Frontiers in Physiology* in 2018, for example, found minimal evidence that electrostimulation yields significant reductions in post-exercise muscle soreness or perceived fatigue.

When discussing high-tech solutions for recovery with my fellow runners, I often remind them that some of the best runners in the world live in Kenya and Ethiopia, comparatively poor countries where athletes have minimal access to things like electrostimulation machines. A close inspection of the lifestyles of these runners shows us what *really* works to promote recovery from training, and it isn't technological wizardry. The best words to describe their overall way of living are *simple* and *slow*. When they're not running, they are generally relaxing. They get plenty of sleep, eat natural foods, and are largely unburdened by modern stressors—such as rush hour, media overload, and consumerism—affecting many denizens of wealthier societies. A case in point is the daily routine of Joshua Cheptegei, who as of this writing holds the men's world records for 5000 and 10,000 meters and who lives and trains with several of his fellow Ugandan elite runners in the sleepy little mountain town of Kapchorwa, close to the Kenyan border:

6:00 a.m.—Run
7:15 a.m.—Breakfast
8:30 a.m.—Rest/nap
10:30 a.m.—Leisure (e.g., board games)
1:00 p.m.—Lunch
2:00 p.m.—Chores/errands
4:30 p.m.—Run
5:00 p.m.—Snack
5:30 p.m.—Rest
8:00 p.m.—Dinner
9:00 p.m.—Bed

As you can see, aside from the runs and the chores, every item on this agenda is restorative in one way or another. It's not just elite African runners who tend not to go in for fancy recovery methods, though. In my experience, pro runners in North America and Europe are—contrary to what you might expect—less prone to make use of electrostimulation machines and the like than are hard-core amateur runners. There's even some evidence that, within the elite ranks, the highest-performing athletes are not as reliant on hifalutin recovery methods as their less

141

successful peers. In her 2019 book *Good to Go*, a comprehensive survey of current athletic recovery methods, science writer Christie Aschwanden reported that, prior to the 2008 Olympics, performance technologist Bill Sands tracked usage of a recovery center at the US Olympic training center. He found that those who spent the most time there were least likely to win a medal in Beijing. To be sure, many pro runners do use fancy recovery methods, but a growing number of experts believe that they function mainly as placebos.

This doesn't mean that such methods are completely without value, but it does mean they are not where the focus of your efforts to promote recovery should be. Instead, your focus should be on the basics of rest, sleep, nutrition, and stress management, just as it is for most professional runners, and for the runners of East Africa especially.

REST

Running creates a need for recovery by inflicting microscopic damage on muscles and other tissues, generating free radicals, producing inflammation, depleting muscle fuel stores, causing dehydration, and fatiguing the nervous system, among other ways. *Not* running—i.e., resting—gives the body an opportunity to address these disruptions and return to homeostasis. Duh, right?

Actually, it's a little more complicated than that. For starters, all rest is not equal. Lying in a hammock and meditating counts as not running, but so does delivering a high-pressure sales presentation at work, and you can be sure that these disparate activities do not have equal recovery value. When the runners of East Africa aren't running, they are generally doing something closer to lying in a hammock than presenting in a board room, and I believe this is part of the reason for their success in the sport. In many other parts of the world, including the United States, where Coach Ben and I live, the lifestyle is quite different, but even pro runners in type A societies like ours try to spend the majority of their non-training time just chilling.

There are exceptions, though, and these individuals prove that you don't have to be or live like a Kenyan to be the best runner you can be. One example is 2016 US Olympian Jared Ward, who works as a statistics instructor at Brigham Young University and is raising four children with his wife, Erica. Needless to say, Jared is a busy man, but he feels strongly that the various roles he juggles in life are complementary, and who can argue otherwise?

The key is to find *some* time for true relaxation every day. Carving out at least twenty minutes for an activity (or form of inactivity) that you enjoy and makes you feel relaxed will give you more recovery benefit than an hour or more of, say, arguing about politics on social media. A study conducted by researchers at Brunel University and published in *Medicine & Science in Sports & Exercise* found that listening to calming music after an exhaustive indoor cycling workout drastically reduced stress hormone levels compared to listening to high-energy music or no music at all. Other good options for relaxation include meditation, reading, journaling, soaking in the tub, having a pleasant conversation with your spouse, and, yes, engaging in relaxing recovery rituals such as wearing progression boots, even though the technologies involved offer little or no recovery benefit in themselves.

Another factor that makes rest a little less simple than merely not running is the relativity of rest. You'll recall from chapter 2 that relative rest entails exercising less than normal, as when a runner who normally runs six miles a day runs only three miles. Relative rest is critical to balancing training and recovery because it allows you to recover while training. Keep in mind that recovery only happens when there is something to recover *from*. A "runner" who never actually runs and *only* rests is not recovering; he's just sedentary. Most of the physiological adaptations that increase fitness are simply extensions of the recovery process—a phenomenon known as supercompensation. Therefore, recovery isn't simply a matter of not running; it's a matter of modulating the training load in a way that creates enough recovery demand to increase fitness while also supplying sufficient recovery opportunity (through absolute rest and relative rest) to steer clear of injury and burnout.

In chapter 3, I introduced the concepts of acute training load (or ATL), which is the combined average volume and intensity of training over the previous week, and chronic training load (or CTL), which is the combined average volume and intensity of training over the past four weeks. Building fitness requires that your ATL exceed your CTL at most times. But getting enough recovery to avoid injury and burnout requires that your ATL not exceed your CTL by more than about 10 percent. The most effective way to keep your acute training load in the optimal zone of 101 to 110 percent of your chronic training load is to practice step cycles, in which your training load increases for two to three weeks and then drops down for one week. This "two or three steps forward, one step back" approach to modulating your training load is how the pros have it both ways: getting fitter while avoiding injury and burnout.

Various apps and websites make it fairly easy to track training loads and ensure you stay between the guardrails of not enough and too much. If you're not especially tech savvy, napkin math can do the job almost as well. If your total training time is up and the fraction of that time spent at higher intensities is the same compared to last week, or if your total training time is the same and the fraction of that time spent at higher intensities is up, then your training load has increased. If the opposite of either of these scenarios is true, your training load has decreased.

There's an even simpler way to stay in the training-load sweet spot, and that's by paying attention to how you feel and reacting accordingly. There are all kinds of glamorous tools, including heart rate variability monitors and sleep monitors, which runners and other athletes may use to assess their recovery status and readiness to train, but research has shown that subjective factors such as mood, motivation, and perceived energy level trump them all. In a 2015 review of existing research in this area, Australian scientists concluded, "Subjective measures reflected acute and chronic training loads with superior sensitivity and consistency than objective measures."

Some professional runners use objective metrics to track their recovery and make decisions about when to rest, but most go by feel, and even those who use objective metrics still allow the subjective measures to have the final say. Two-time World Cross Country Championships qualifier Neely Gracey is typical in this regard. "If I need a day off or a day on the bike instead of a run, I take it," she said in one interview. It takes a combination of experience and mindfulness to learn how to read your body's (and mind's) signals well enough to know when it's okay to push ahead and when you need to dial back, but if you make the effort, there's really no better guide.

SLEEP

One of the biggest myths about professional runners is that they sleep a lot.

Just kidding. Pro runners really do sleep a lot! I saw this firsthand during the three months I spent living in the home of NAZ Elite member Matt Llano (who has since left the team). Matt typically slept nine to ten hours at night and another one to two hours in the afternoon. By the time I left Flagstaff, I understood why. Napping is not a part of my normal lifestyle, but toward the end of my stint as a fake pro runner, I reluctantly took up the habit. I really had no choice—when my training load passed a certain threshold (around eighty-five miles of running per week), I simply couldn't get through the afternoon without catching a few winks. Needless to say, even my heaviest weeks of training under Coach Ben were substantially lighter than those that Matt and his teammates were absorbing, so you can imagine how much more urgent their need for sleep was.

It stands to reason that increased training loads heighten the body's sleep requirements. In the previous section, I mentioned that there are different degrees of rest. Sleep, of course, represents the highest degree of rest. With the possible exception of the first hour or so after a run, when the body returns from an exertional state to homeostasis, more recovery occurs during sleep than at any other time. The consequences for runners of not getting enough sleep are severe. A 2020 study conducted by Tunisian scientists and published in *Physiology & Behavior* found that reducing sleep from eight hours to four hours for just one night increased perceived effort and re-duced self-selected pace in a run the next morning. Findings like these should be a wake-up call, so to speak, if you are among the majority of nonelite runners who operate in a state of chronic, mild sleep deprivation.

Although it is well established that sleep needs increase with training loads, there is no universal formula you can use to determine how much sleep you need based on your current training load. Sleep requirements are highly individual and therefore must be assessed subjectively. If you feel refreshed when you get out of bed in the morning and you don't feel sleepy again until you're just about ready to climb back into bed at night, you're getting enough sleep; otherwise you're probably not.

The best way to ensure you consistently get enough sleep is to create habits around it. Sleep experts offer the following tips for developing an effective sleep routine:

- Go to bed and wake up at the same time every day, even on weekends.
- Make sure your bedroom is dark, quiet, and comfortable.
- Perform a relaxing ritual before going to bed (more on this later in the chapter).
- Banish all screens (phone, television, computer) from your bedroom.
- Avoid exercising and consuming alcohol and caffeine late in the day if these things seem to interfere with your sleep.
- Consider experimenting with a natural sleep-promoting supplement such as melatonin, GABA, valerian, CBD oil, kava, passionflower, glycine, chamomile, 5-HTP, or magnesium, but do your research first.

Establishing better sleep habits can be difficult insofar as it requires breaking existing habits. I recommend a thirty-day challenge as a way to overcome the inertia of any current habits you need to break. Make a conscious commitment to stick with your plan for getting more and better sleep for thirty days, no excuses. This should be enough time to get some momentum behind the new habits so that less effort is required to maintain them.

146

STRESS MANAGEMENT

You may have noticed that I've avoided using the term *overtraining* in this book, choosing *burnout* instead. The reason is that I find *overtraining* to be misleading because it erroneously suggests that too much training is the sole cause of the underperformance and fatigue that characterize the condition it refers to. In reality, burnout (as I insist on calling it) is caused by stress, of which training is just one form. The key to avoiding burnout, therefore, is managing total stress, or *allostatic load* as science calls it. Not training too much is certainly one way to achieve this objective, and so are getting adequate rest and sleep, but in addition to these measures there are stress-management skills you can develop to help yourself handle your training better.

A study led by Frank Perna of Boston University School of Medicine and published in the *Annals of Behavioral Medicine* in 2003 looked at the effect of one particular stress-management method—cognitive behavioral therapy—on stress, mood, and illness and injury rates in college rowers. Thirty-four male and female rowers were split evenly into two groups and monitored for three months after one group received cognitive behavioral therapy and the other did not. During the three-month follow-up period, members of the treatment group were found to have missed nearly 80 percent fewer days of training due to illness or injury than members of the control group. Levels of negative affect (i.e., low mood) and cortisol, a stress hormone, were also significantly reduced in the treatment group.

In the summer I spent with NAZ Elite, I was profoundly impressed by how well the team's individual members managed stress. It's one of several shared psychological traits that I didn't expect to observe but couldn't possibly miss. These young athletes kept stress at bay primarily through their thinking style, which is exactly what cognitive behavioral therapy aims to retrain, and which I will discuss in depth in chapter 9. But they did it in other ways, too, such as by actively maintaining a healthy run/life balance, by seeking out the services of team sports psychologist Shannon Thompson, and, in the case of at least one runner (Scott Fauble), by meditating regularly.

147

Because I lived with him, I was able to study Matt Llano's stress-management habits closely. More high-strung than most of his teammates, Matt made overt efforts to decompress and maintain his equanimity. One way he did so was by spending quality time with his dog, Harlow, which he adopted not long before I came to stay with him. Matt ran with her, cuddled with her, and took her out to romp in local parks and lakes, and her salutary effect on his psyche was unmistakable.

Another way in which Matt managed stress effectively was by tinkering in his garage and doing crafts of different sorts. For example, toward the end of my time in Flagstaff, Matt spent a few days creating a piece of string art for his friend Alicia, painstakingly spelling out the name of her new baby (Skylar) with string and pegs on a wooden board. Watching him work, I could see how centering it was for him to channel his creativity and his affection into this outlet.

Somewhat reclusive by nature, Matt also made a point of getting out and socializing for the sake of his mental well-being. Every other Friday or so, for instance, he would visit the home of teammate Aaron Braun and his wife, Annika, to play Scrabble or some other game, a ritual he inaugurated at the urging of Coach Ben, who reminded Matt that sometimes the best thing you can do for your running is to get away from running.

All of these measures—enjoying a pet, being creative, doing nice things for other people, and socializing and playing games—are scientifically proven to reduce stress. If you want to boost your recovery capacity and your running by managing stress like a pro, you could do a lot worse than to follow Matt Llano's example.

NUTRITION

When you think about nutrition for post-run recovery, the first thing you think of, in all likelihood, is supplements such as protein powders and CBD. That's because supplement makers have poured gobs of money into marketing, advertising, and research in order to create this association in your mind. This well-bankrolled blizzard of messaging disguises the fact that real food has a much greater impact on recovery than any supplement. Unfortunately, real food lacks a huge marketing budget to make its case (when's the last time you saw an advertisement for spinach?), but in recent years, scientists have finally gotten around to studying its effects on athletic recovery. A study conducted by Brazilian researchers and published in *Biology of Sport* in 2018, for example, found that two weeks of increased fruit and vegetable consumption improved total antioxidant capacity (a key recovery mechanism) in triathletes.

Rare is the East African elite runner who takes recovery supplements. Granted, this is largely because supplements are hard to find in their part of the world, but nevertheless it demonstrates that supplements aren't needed to recover well enough to run at the highest level. Indeed, the few supplements, including branched-chain amino acids, that *have* been shown to enhance recovery processes offer nothing more than the nutrients found in the kinds of natural foods that make up the Kenyan and Ethiopian diets. What's more, a sizable fraction of pro runners living in areas where recovery supplements are widely available don't use them either. Many avoid such products for fear of unwittingly ingesting ingredients that might trigger a positive drug test, but if supplements were truly needed to optimize recovery, you can be sure that a lot more pro runners would take a chance on them.

If you're wondering what you should eat for breakfast, lunch, and dinner to optimize your recovery from training, don't. The meals you eat as a runner need to serve a variety of functions beyond aiding recovery—such as supporting overall health, reducing injury risk, fueling your runs, and promoting a lean body composition. It would be a mistake to tailor your diet to just one function. Fortunately, the same set of eating habits that serve to optimize muscle recovery are also best for the other important jobs that a runner's diet needs to do. I will share these habits in the next chapter.

Where recovery is concerned, it's not just what you eat but *when* that matters. Nutrients from food provide the raw materials needed to carry out many recovery processes: protein to repair damaged muscles, carbohydrate to refuel them, water to restore blood volume, and certain fats and antioxidants to modulate inflammation. If you

149

go too long without eating and drinking at any point during the day—but especially in the first couple of hours after a run—you will compromise your recovery.

This was shown in a study on the effects of intermittent fasting on endurance performance. Researchers from the University of Malaysia had ten subjects complete a test of anaerobic capacity and a time-to-exhaustion test on stationary bikes every other day throughout a ten-day period of intermittent fasting (which simply entailed skipping lunch). Meanwhile, ten control subjects who ate the same number of calories each day but did not skip lunch completed the same series of tests. As expected, the controls performed consistently in these tests. Members of the intermittent fasting group, on the other hand, experienced a sharp initial drop in performance that they only partially recovered from after ten days. The authors of the study, which was published in the *European Journal of Sport Science* in 2018, attributed this performance dip to impaired recovery resulting from the long gap between meals.

Getting appropriate nutrition relatively soon after training is especially important on days when you exercise more than once, as the pros do most days. In a 2017 review published in *Sports Medicine*, Danielle McCartney and colleagues at Griffith University reported that consuming adequate amounts of carbohydrate and water after an initial workout improved performance in a second workout completed later the same day by 4 percent. This effect was blunted, however, when subjects ate a meal two to four hours before the first workout instead of starting it in a fasted state, indicating that optimal recovery depends on eating appropriately *before* you exercise, not just after.

There's no need to get overly scientific about your eating schedule. Other research has yielded evidence that athletes tend to recover just fine if they simply eat breakfast, lunch, and dinner on a normal schedule and add a snack or two if and when they become hungry between meals. Here, too, East Africa's elite runners validate science. Like Joshua Cheptegei, most of these athletes train in camps, and in the camp environment everyone eats on the same, unvarying schedule. In Kenya, the standard routine is an early breakfast of milky tea before the morning run; a large second breakfast, usually featuring chapati (a type of bread similar to naan) immediately afterward; a lunch comprising some combination of rice, beans, potatoes, and greens before the afternoon run; a dinner centered on ugali (a classic Kenyan staple best described as a dense corn-flour cake); and fruit and water throughout the day as desired.

You needn't get too scientific about the composition of your post-run meals and snacks either, as was demonstrated by a famous 2015 study in which a fast-food meal eaten after an intense cycling session was found to have the same effect on performance in a subsequent time trial as a mixture of energy bars and specially formulated recovery beverages. This does not mean you should start eating cheeseburgers after runs, as there are other factors to consider, including your long-term health, but it does underscore the point that everyday foods will do the trick.

CORRECTIVE EXERCISE

The term *corrective exercise* sounds like a form of punishment, kind of like *reform school*. In fact, though, it refers to therapeutic exercises done for the sake of addressing limitations in flexibility, mobility, and strength that compromise an athlete's ability to perform sports movements, thereby reducing efficiency and increasing injury risk. Corrective exercise is not a specific type of activity, like Pilates, but instead encompasses all types of activity—static stretches, dynamic stretches, foam rolling, bodyweight strength exercises, and more—that serve this basic purpose. It's also not a recovery method in the usual sense of facilitating the restoration of physiological homeostasis after running, but I still like to think of it as a recovery modality because it acts to reverse some of the negative effects that running has on the body, such as creating tight spots in the muscles, and also because it's relaxing.

Most nonelite runners eschew corrective exercise either because they aren't aware of its existence or because they would rather devote their limited time to something they perceive as more important. If you were not previously aware of the existence of corrective exercise,

151

well, you are now. As to the second excuse for not doing it, I have two responses:

First, it works! Consider your feet, a part of the runner's anatomy that doesn't get enough attention. A 2020 study led by Brazilian researchers and published in the *American Journal of Sports Medicine* reported that a corrective exercise routine for the feet reduced the injury rate by 41 percent in a group of eighteen runners (half of whom served as controls). Imagine two out of every five injuries in your running career never happening—*that's* what a bit of daily corrective exercise can do for you.

The second thing I have to say in favor of corrective exercise is that it's easy to incorporate into your day. Most professional runners have some kind of daily corrective exercise routine they do right at home with little or no equipment and no need to shower afterward. Champion ultrarunner Rob Krar, for example, starts each day with a series of active isolated stretches involving an elastic strap. I like to do my own routine right before bed, as a way to wind down.

The specific exercises I do have been recommended to me by physical therapists to address my individual needs. It's best that you, too, adopt a corrective exercise routine that is tailored to your needs, as no two runners have exactly the same collection of tight spots, weaknesses, and imbalances. There are, however, many exercises that can't hurt and are likely to help most runners because they address issues that are nearly universal in runners' bodies. I'll conclude this chapter by presenting a selection of these corrective exercises that will hold you over until you develop a custom routine with the help of a physical therapist.

Kneeling Hip Flexor Stretch

Most runners lack sufficient hip-flexion range of motion. This stretch lengthens the hip flexors.

Kneel on your right knee and place your left foot flat on the floor with a ninety-degree bend in the knee. Grab the ends of a strap in both hands, loop it around your left knee and pull gently toward your body. Keeping your torso upright, contract your glutes and press your hips forward until you feel a good stretch at the front of your right hip. Hold the stretch for one minute and then reverse your stance and stretch the left hip.

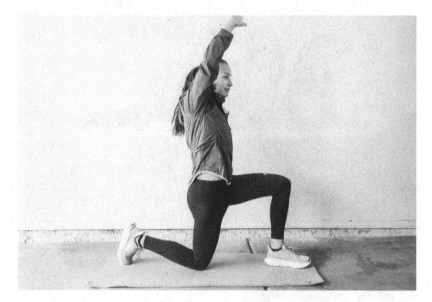

153

IT Band Foam Rolling

The iliotibial bands, which are long tendons that run along the outer side of the thighs, are another area that tends to be overly tight in most runners. Stretching doesn't do much for them, but foam rolling does.

Lie on your right side with your right forearm propping up your torso and your right leg resting on the foam roller just below the hip socket. Slowly roll your outer thigh back and forth over the roller. After thirty seconds or so, flip over and work the left IT band.

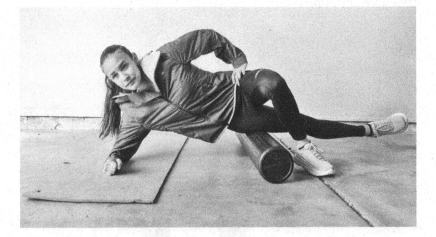

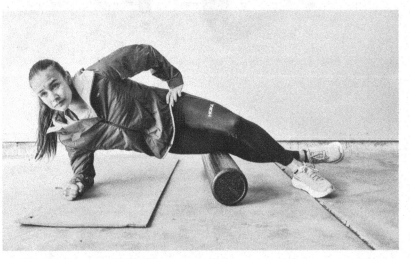

Isometric Hip Adduction with Foam Roller

In many people, the hip abductors (the muscles on the inner side of the thighs) are too weak to properly perform their job of stabilizing the pelvis during running. I learned this method of strengthening them from AJ Gregg at HYPO2 in Flagstaff, who along with his brother, Wes, serves as a strength coach to NAZ Elite.

Lie faceup on the floor with your knees bent sharply and your feet on the floor about eight inches apart. Position a foam roller between your knees. Now press your knees together as though you're trying to crush the foam roller and hold the contraction for ten seconds. Relax for five seconds and repeat ten times.

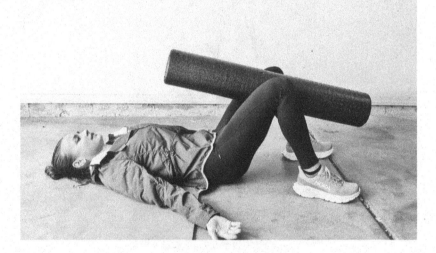

Single-Leg Balance

Balancing barefoot on one foot with your eyes closed is a simple and effective way to strengthen important stabilizing muscles in the lower leg and foot that are neglected in shod running.

Stand barefoot on your right foot, close your eyes, and count to thirty. If you lose your balance, try again, restarting the count at zero. Once you've succeeded in balancing for thirty seconds, repeat the exercise on your left foot.

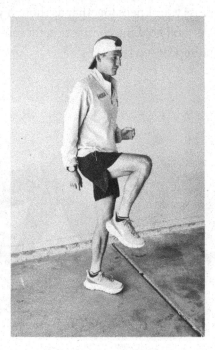

Wall Ankle Mobilization

This test of ankle mobility doubles as a way to increase ankle mobility by stretching the Achilles tendons and calf muscles.

Stand facing a wall with the toes of one foot positioned a few inches from it. Without raising your heel from the floor, bend your knee and tap the wall with your kneecap. Now slide the foot back a couple of inches and tap the wall with your kneecap again. Keep moving back little by little until you can no longer tap the wall without raising your heel. You'll feel an increasing stretch in your Achilles tendon as you go. Now repeat with the other leg.

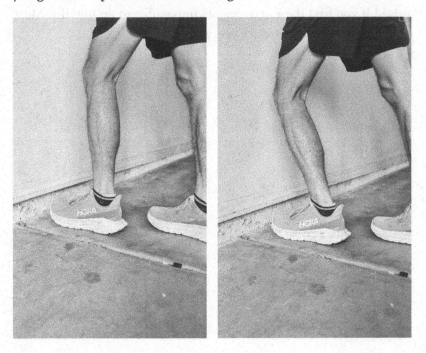

Toe Yoga

The big toes play an underappreciated role in aligning, stabilizing, and propelling the body during running. Chances are you have less strength in, and less control over, your big toes than you should. This surprisingly challenging exercise will fix the issue over time.

Stand normally on a hard surface in bare feet. Try to lift the big toe of your right foot while keeping your other toes in contact with the floor. Pause for one second and then press your big toe down to the floor and raise your other toes, again holding for one second. Repeat several times and then do the same with your left foot. Don't be surprised if you find these movements impossible to do initially. Most runners do, but with practice everyone improves.

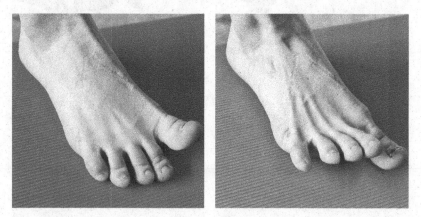

MATT FITZGERALD AND BEN ROSARIO

Coach's Tip

Run/Life Balance

Like many runners, I learned to respect recovery the hard way—by paying the price for *not* respecting it. The process began in high school when, as an obsessed athlete, I valued my sleep over nearly everything else in my life. I would stop studying at exactly nine o'clock to go to bed, regardless of what I had left to do, and my grades suffered accordingly. I skipped my senior prom to ensure I would get enough rest before the district track meet, and my relationship with my girlfriend suffered accordingly. I took fast food completely out of my diet in my junior and senior years, and—well, maybe that was for the best. The point is, as amateur runners, we need to value our recovery yet balance it with the other important things in our life.

As a college freshman, I swung way too far toward the other end of the spectrum. I partied. A lot. I pulled an all-nighter. I chased girls. I reintroduced fast food to my diet, making more 3:00 a.m. drive-through missions than I care to recall. Did I mention I partied a lot? And yes, my running suffered accordingly. So I am speaking from experience on the need for balance in one's life. I wish I could say I found that balance in my sophomore year, but it was more that I swung back to how I approached things in high school, with occasional forays into my freshman ways during the off-season. But in college, your body can do things it just cannot do ten or fifteen years later. Hungover twenty-milers, a diet of ramen noodles and frozen pizza (the cheap kind), and video game marathons are not really what I would suggest for someone who's serious about running, and yet I pulled off some decent performances in those days.

So that's the hard way to learn what does and doesn't work for recovery as a runner. The easy way is to model your recovery habits after the pros. The NAZ Elite runners are true professionals in this regard. Having worked with them every day for the past eight years, I can tell you with 100 percent conviction that it all begins with **sleep**. I believe the human body craves consistency in general, but in sleep especially. The sleep-expert tips Matt shared in the preceding chapter were all things I know to have worked either for myself, for my athletes, or both. I know that Scott Fauble meditates before bed to be completely relaxed. Stephanie Bruce has a bedtime and she sticks to it. For me, reading before bed has always led to a better night's sleep than watching television.

As Matt points out, though, sleep needs are highly individual, and therefore so too are optimal sleep habits. On our team, we have athletes who take a nap at the same time every single day, we have one athlete who takes a nap whenever the mood strikes—even if that's at 6:00 p.m.—and we have one athlete who may never have taken a nap in her entire life. And yet they have all achieved an incredible amount of success.

For recovery, a close second to sleep in importance is **stress management**. I have often used the phrase "A happy runner is a fit runner." We know that money can't buy happiness; nor can running be the singular path to our emotional well-being. I have met many a sad runner and, on a more serious level, many a depressed runner. Yes, I am coming back to balance again. I was so unbalanced as a young athlete. I vividly remember staying up all night after a disappointing indoor 5000-meter race in Ames, Iowa, lamenting my performance, envisioning what I could do to improve, wanting so badly to go back in time and start the race over. At twenty years old, running eighty miles a week, with a resting heart rate of forty beats per minute, I seemed a beacon of health, and yet, I was unhealthy. My stress was running-related, while perhaps your stress is work-related. Perhaps it is family-related. We all have stress. It's unavoidable. That's why it's called stress *management*.

If you are serious about your running, as I would assume you are as a reader of this book, then you also ought to be serious about managing your stress. It might not seem particularly running-related, but I can promise that reducing the stress in your life will put you in a position to be a better runner. That is a Coach Ben guarantee. Having worked with elite athletes for more than a decade, I know for a fact that those who work on this part of their life see the work pay off in their running. I'll step down from my soapbox before I stray above my pay grade, but before I do, let me just say this: please seek help for stress if and when you need it. Go to your friends. Share your thoughts and feelings with your significant other, or with a family member. And, of course, seek help from a professional if necessary. All of these resources can lead to better stress management.

Close behind stress management, **nutrition** and **corrective exercise** are equally important in recovery, but I will focus on corrective exercise here before moving on to nutrition in the next chapter. Although most runners don't associate corrective exercise with recovery, I've seen this method produce tangible results. Our team's strength and conditioning coaches, AJ and Wes Gregg, have saved our bacon many times by getting athletes on a corrective exercise routine unique to their individual needs. Back in my day, it was throw some ice on it, pop a couple of ibuprofen, and hope it goes away. Now, when you add it all up, professional athletes are spending several hours a week on exercises to correct imbalances, to heal injuries, to prevent injuries, and to enhance performance.

Do amateur runners have that kind of time? Probably not, but Matt has given you six simple exercises that amount to a routine of no longer than ten minutes. We're talking about seventy minutes over the course of a week. That seems doable, doesn't it? (Remember, his examples are meant simply to hold you over until a physical therapist can tailor a routine specifically to you.)

My parting thought on the topic of recovery is that, more than any particular method, it's the attitude that professional runners have toward recovery that sets them apart. In a word, they *respect* it in a way that I did not until I paid the full price for not respecting it. They understand that their running can only ever be as good as their recovery, and this is as true for you as it is for them.

161

EAT LIKE A PRO

*I*T'S NOT SURPRISING THAT professional runners everywhere train similarly. After all, we know that training has a huge impact on performance and that some training methods work better than others. The sport of running has become so competitive at the elite level that even the most gifted athlete can't hope to reach the top without making use of the best methods, so it's really only to be expected that elite runners in all corners of the globe adhere to the same training principles and methods.

What about diet, though? Like training, food has a significant impact on running performance. Also like training, diet can either help or hinder a runner depending on the specific practices chosen. Shouldn't we therefore expect pro runners everywhere to have converged on a single, optimal way of eating, just as they've converged on a single, optimal way of training?

At first glance, this would appear impossible on a global scale. Different cultures around the world have diverse ways of eating, and the runners in those disparate environments tend to eat in ways that are consistent with their culture, hence differently from one another. In the preceding chapter, I mentioned that Kenya's elite runners eat a lot of ugali. Nowhere else in the world will you find this dish on the plates of elite runners (or nonrunners, for that matter). If eating the same way means eating the same *foods*, then it's obvious professional runners don't all eat the same way.

If, on the other hand, we accept a broader definition of eating the same way, we come to another conclusion altogether. In Ethiopia, for example, a type of bread called injera occupies a place in the diet that is almost identical to that of ugali in the Kenyan diet, and it's nutritionally very similar: a whole-grain food that's high in starch, fiber, vitamins, minerals, and antioxidants. For many Asian pro runners, rice is the dietetic equivalent of ugali and injera, and for many South American pro runners, it's potatoes. Name any region or country you like, in fact, and you will find that one or more starchy natural foods serve as staples in the diet of elite runners there.

The point I'm trying to make with these examples is that *ways of eating* are best defined not by specific foods but rather by underlying patterns. While professional runners don't all eat the same foods, by and large they do share a set of underlying eating habits. I know this because I literally wrote the book on how elite endurance athletes eat.

In 2015, I traveled all over the world to dine with and study the diets of elite endurance athletes. I shared tables with Dutch cyclists, Brazilian triathletes, Kenyan runners, Japanese runners, and Canadian cross-country skiers. I also created a diet survey that was completed by elite athletes representing a wide range of endurance disciplines in more than forty countries. What I discovered through this very fun research process was that, underneath superficial differences in the specific foods they eat, elite endurance athletes in all disciplines and in every part of the world practice the same five core eating habits. Formulated as rules (because what's a diet without rules?), these habits are as follows:

1. Eat everything.
2. Eat quality.
3. Eat carb-centered.
4. Eat enough.
5. Eat individually.

I believe these five habits constitute the optimal diet for all endurance athletes, including nonprofessional runners like you and me. By adopting them, you will actualize the full potential benefit of nutrition for health, fitness, and performance. You'll have plenty of energy for runs, get fitter faster, recover well from your workouts, minimize your risk of getting sick or injured, optimize your body composition for running, and limit the likelihood of burning out. Best of all, adhering to the core eating habits of the world's best runners is easy—much easier than sticking with most popular diets.

EAT EVERYTHING

The reason most popular diets are hard to stick with is that they're based on avoidance. The paleo diet forbids grains and dairy; plant-based diets eliminate meat, fish, dairy, and eggs; ketogenic diets strictly limit all carbohydrate-rich foods; and so on. By contrast, most professional runners go out of their way to maintain a well-rounded and inclusive diet that incorporates all types of foods.

Each food type is nutritionally distinct from the others. Vegetables are richer in many vitamins and minerals than any other food type, for example, while meat and fish contain more and higher-quality protein than any other food type. Eating everything ensures that the overall diet is balanced and free of deficiencies. Such nutritional well-roundedness is helpful to anyone interested in good health, as has been shown in epidemiological studies going as far back as the 1970s. More recently, Harvard researchers reported in the *Journal of Nutrition* in 2015 that, within a population of 7,470 adults, the rate of metabolic syndrome was significantly lower among those who scored highest on the US healthy food diversity index. A varied diet is even more helpful to runners, who, in seeking not just health but also fitness and performance, place extra demands on their metabolism through their training. Runners who go down the avoidance path all too often get into trouble when training stress exposes deficiencies created by the lack of variety in their eating.

Take Julie Benson, a runner from my native New Hampshire whose story I shared in *The Endurance Diet*. In the hope of improving her marathon time, Julie allowed herself to be talked into trying the popular no-sugar no-grains (NSNG) diet. Alas, instead of getting faster, she came apart. Tired all day every day, she felt lousy in even her easiest runs, and her workout performances cratered. After hanging on for several weeks to see if her body would eventually adapt to her new way of eating (it didn't), Julie went back to eating everything, and her running immediately rebounded.

It bears mentioning that not a single member of NAZ Elite was on any kind of avoidance diet while I was with the team, with the lone exception of Stephanie Bruce, who is allergic to dairy, soy, and eggs and has celiac disease and therefore can't eat wheat or other gluten-containing foods. Yet even she went out of her way to eat as diversely as possible within her individual constraints.

EAT QUALITY

If "eating everything" has left you with the impression that pro runners follow an "anything goes" diet—well, they don't. In fact, like all health-conscious eaters, professional runners have very high standards for their diet. Unlike most popular diets, however, where the governing standards are all about avoiding certain types of food or nutrients, the diet favored by professional runners and other elite endurance athletes is characterized by standards of *quality* that are applied across all food types.

In nutrition science, "quality" has a specific meaning. Simply put, a particular type of food is considered to be high quality if eating it tends to be associated with positive health outcomes such as reduced chronic disease risk and a lower mortality rate. Low-quality food types are just the opposite: foods that tend to be associated with negative health outcomes. The highest-quality food types are vegetables, fruits, nuts and seeds, whole grains, and seafood. Unprocessed meat and dairy are also generally associated with positive health outcomes, though not to the same degree. Processed food types such as refined grains, processed meats, sweets, fried foods, and other foods containing added fats are all associated with negative health outcomes, so they're classified as low-quality.

Nutrition scientists have come up with various indices for scoring diet quality. Among these are the Healthy Eating Index and the Mediterranean Diet Quality Index. Although these tools were created for

165

the purpose of supporting health-based dietary choices, fitness rests on a foundation of health, so it comes as no surprise that research has also uncovered an association between diet quality and fitness-related outcomes.

A good example of this research is a study published in the *Journal of Sports Medicine and Physical Fitness* in 2019. Researchers at the University of Bergamo recruited forty college athletes, including twenty runners, and separated them into two groups. Members of one group received nutritional counseling intended to promote adherence to a Mediterranean-type diet centered on the consumption of vegetables, fruits, herbs, nuts, beans, poultry, seafood, and dairy, while those in the other group were allowed to continue eating as usual. Both groups trained normally and were monitored for three months. Before and after this three-month period, all forty subjects underwent physiological testing. Runners who received nutritional counseling and adhered to a high-quality Mediterranean diet showed significantly greater improvements in VO_2max and body composition than runners who stuck with their existing eating habits.

Another study that was conducted around the same time by a different research team found that the performance benefits of a high-quality diet begin to manifest a lot sooner than three months—at least if you're switching over from a low-quality Western diet. Researchers at Saint Louis University invited eleven recreational runners to complete a pair of 5K time trials, one after four days on a high-quality Mediterranean diet and another after four days on a low-quality Western diet. On average, the subjects ran 6 percent faster (equivalent to ninety seconds) when fueled by the Mediterranean diet. Lead author Edward Weiss said of these results in an interview for *Science Daily*, "This study provides evidence that a diet that is known to be good for health is also good for exercise performance."

I'm not suggesting that every runner should follow a Mediterranean diet. My message, rather, is that every runner who wishes to gain the greatest possible performance benefit from food should maintain a high-quality diet that features plenty of vegetables, fruit, nuts and seeds, healthy oils (e.g., olive oil), whole grains, dairy, seafood, and unprocessed meat, while limiting the amounts of refined

166

grains, processed meats, sweets, and foods with added fats (including fried foods).

A number of years ago, I created my own diet quality index especially for endurance athletes. Much simpler than the various scientific instruments used to assess diet quality, the Diet Quality Score (DQS) is intended to make it easy for athletes to monitor and regulate their diet quality from day to day. You can find complete information on what's included in each food category, how to judge portion sizes, and how scoring works on my website racingweight.com. There's also a DQS smartphone app available in iPhone and Android versions.

EAT CARB-CENTERED

No diet fad has done more harm to more runners in recent years than the various low-carb diets, including the low-carb high-fat (LCHF) diet and the keto diet. Despite all the chest-thumping you see on social media from runners claiming to be delighted with the results of their low-carb diet, the vast majority of runners who go down this road are disappointed with the results. For starters, it's a highly restrictive way of eating that drains much of the enjoyment out of the food experience. It also fosters a toxic fear- and guilt-based relationship with food that is unpleasant in the best cases and leads to full-blown eating disorders in the worst cases.

On a physical level, the more extreme low-carb diets are highly unbalanced nutritionally and may result in serious negative health consequences over the long term. Evidence of this comes from a 2019 study led by Sara Seidelmann of Brigham and Women's Hospital. Her team analyzed diet and mortality data from more than 15,400 middle-age men and women who were tracked over a period of twenty-five years as part of the Atherosclerosis Risk in Communities (ARIC) study. The main finding of the study, as reported in the *Lancet Public Health* in August 2018, was that subjects who got less than 40 percent of their daily calories from carbs died four years younger, on average, than those who got between 40 and 70 percent of their calories from carbs. The problem appeared to be that people who reduced their carbohydrate intake replaced those calories with low-quality alternatives.

167

Specifically, men and women who replaced carbs with large amounts of animal-derived fat or protein tended to die younger, whereas those who picked plant-based substitutes (like nuts) did not.

Much more research needs to be done before it can be firmly concluded that long-term adherence to a low-carb diet puts one's health at risk. In the meantime, it is already well established that low-carb diets are harmful to endurance performance. The purported benefit of cutting carbs as a runner is that it forces the body to rely more on fat to fuel runs, which over time increases the fat-burning capacity of the muscles. Because the body stores vastly greater amounts of fat fuel than carbohydrate fuel, this adaptation is believed to boost endurance. Science has demonstrated that training on a low-carb diet does indeed increase the fat-burning capacity of the muscles. However, this benefit comes at a huge cost: a commensurate reduction in the carbohydrate-burning capacity of the muscles that results in a net negative effect of carb-cutting on running performance.

The crux of the issue is that fat is a very inefficient fuel, requiring a lot more oxygen than carbohydrate-derived fuels (namely glycogen and glucose) to metabolize, and there's a fixed limit on how much oxygen a given runner can consume—quantified as VO_2max. You can't just absorb more oxygen beyond your normal limit to make up for the fact that your low-carb diet has made your muscles more dependent on fat fuel, which yields less energy and less speed per unit of oxygen consumed. As a result, this dependency on fat essentially deprives you of your highest running gears, causing you to hit your maximum rate of oxygen consumption at a lower speed.

Some of the best research on the consequences of low-carb eating on endurance performance has been done by Louise Burke and colleagues at the Australian Institute of Sport. In one experiment, Burke's team recruited twenty-six elite race walkers to serve as subjects and separated them into two groups, one of which was placed on a high-carb diet (8.6 grams per kilogram of body weight daily) while the other adhered to a ketogenic diet (less than 50 total grams of carbs daily) throughout a twenty-five-day period of intensified training. Physiological testing and performance testing were done on both groups before and after the intervention.

In an earlier version of the same experiment, the second performance test came immediately after the athletes in the keto group completed the "fat adaptation" process. However, critics objected that this protocol did not reflect the way ketogenic diets are practiced in the real world, where savvier athletes allow themselves time to replenish their muscle glycogen stores through carbohydrate loading prior to competition. In response to this critique, Burke's team made an adjustment in the follow-up study, permitting the unlucky race walkers who'd been placed on the keto diet to top off their muscle glycogen stores by eating more carbs for seventeen days ahead of the second round of testing. In principle, this extra step enabled them to have the best of both worlds, retaining the increased fat-burning capacity they'd earned through carbohydrate restriction without being compromised by low muscle carbohydrate stores on "race" day.

As expected, the keto diet achieved its objective of increasing fat-burning capacity in the athletes who followed it, their peak rate of fat oxidation during exercise jumping from 0.6 gram/minute to 1.3 grams/minute over the course of the twenty-five-day intervention and staying elevated throughout the replenishment period that followed. However, as in the first experiment, this seemingly beneficial adaptation was not really beneficial at all, resulting in a sharp increase in the energy cost of walking at race speeds. On average, performance in a 10K racewalk declined by an average of 2.3 percent in the athletes who had done the keto diet while improving by 4.8 percent among athletes who followed a high-carb diet straight through.

Many other studies have produced similar findings, so it's no wonder that elite runners never jumped aboard the low-carb bandwagon. Although habitual carbohydrate intake levels vary widely from place to place, it's high even in those places with the lowest intake, ranging from 60 percent of daily calories in the Netherlands, according to one study, to 78 percent of daily calories in Ethiopia, according to another. Most runners are able to perform equally well at any level within this range provided their diet is high in overall quality. I saw this for myself in 2015 when I traveled to Kenya to run a marathon and conduct research for my book. Throughout my two-week stay, I ate traditional Kenyan foods exclusively, my carb intake increasing from 60 percent of daily calories to 75 percent in the process. I felt no difference in my energy level, performed well in the marathon, and even lost a couple of pounds.

Based on the totality of this information, I recommend that non-elite runners aim to get roughly 60 percent of their daily calories from carbohydrate as a baseline during periods of race-focused training. This is not difficult to do. The typical Western diet is slightly less than 50 percent carbohydrate. By simply shifting your eating toward high-quality food types, which tend to be more carb-rich than many commonly eaten low-quality foods, you will boost your overall carbohydrate intake above the 60 percent threshold. There's no need to pull out your calculator. Just try to center most of your meals and snacks on a high-quality, high-carb food. Here's an example of a day's worth of pro-style, high-quality, carb-centered eating:

BREAKFAST
Whole-grain granola
Plain Greek yogurt
Fresh raspberries
Coffee

SNACK
Banana and sugar-free peanut butter

LUNCH
Brown rice
Stir-fried vegetables
Tofu
Tomato juice

SNACK
Avocado toast

DINNER
Broiled salmon
Steamed broccoli florets

Roasted red potatoes
White wine
Dark chocolate

Getting even more than 60 percent of your daily calories from carbs won't hurt you and may even yield additional benefits during especially heavy periods of training. Elite ultrarunner Jim Walmsley is among the many pro runners who intentionally increase their carb intake when they're really piling on the miles.

Some professional runners intentionally reduce their carb intake on rest days and during breaks from formal training as a weight-management technique, and it's okay to emulate this practice as a nonelite runner. A growing number of pro runners also do occasional *depletion runs*, which are runs performed under conditions of carbo-hydrate restriction. Like low-carb diets, depletion runs boost the fat-burning capacity of the muscles. Unlike low-carb diets, however, depletion runs offer this benefit without reducing carbohydrate-burning capacity, VO_2max, training tolerance, and running economy. In fact, depletion runs are proven to *increase* VO_2max by activating particular genes involved in aerobic metabolism.

The simplest way to practice depletion runs is to do a longer, low-intensity run on an empty stomach first thing in the morning, consuming water only or water plus electrolytes (but no carbs) during the run. A somewhat fancier, research-backed protocol entails doing a normally fueled high-intensity interval run in the afternoon, eating a very low-carb dinner afterward, sleeping, and then doing an easy run on an empty stomach first thing in the morning.

If you choose to incorporate depletion runs into your training, pro-ceed cautiously and don't overdo them. For example, if your normal long-run distance is fifteen miles, start with a ten-mile carb-restricted long run and go from there. One depletion run every week to two weeks is plenty. Keep in mind that they are just one tool among many that will aid your running when sprinkled into the training process in judicious amounts.

EAT ENOUGH

In wealthy countries like the United States, people tend to be more concerned about eating too much than about not eating enough, and with good reason. Nearly three in four Americans over the age of twenty are overweight or obese. For runners, though, the consequences of not eating enough are actually more severe than those of eating too much.

Running attenuates the various health risks associated with overeating, including high blood pressure, insulin resistance, and hyperlipidemia. This is in no way a "get out of jail free" card with respect to the health consequences of eating too much, but the only significant *performance* penalty of eating too much is the higher energy cost of running with extra body weight. Compare this to the known consequences of eating too little as a runner: low energy, loss of muscle mass, reduced performance, slower post-run recovery, lower metabolic rate, attenuated fitness gains, and increased risk of injury and illness. Simply put, if you eat too much, you're likely to arrive on the start line of your next race a few pounds over your optimal competition weight, but if you eat too little, you're unlikely to make it to the start line of your next race *period*.

Professional runners rarely make the mistake of eating too little. It's easy to understand why when you look at what happens when an athlete at the elite level does go down this path. Molly Seidel is a great example. As a junior at Notre Dame University, Molly was the surprise winner of the NCAA championships 10,000 meters. The pressure she subsequently felt to live up to the standard she'd set for herself led her to reduce her food intake, which in turn resulted in multiple stress fractures. Although Molly won three more NCAA titles before graduating, she was ultimately forced to take a long hiatus from competitive running and seek treatment for disordered eating. By 2020, Molly was back to eating enough and back on form, finishing second behind NAZ Elite's Aliphine Tuliamuk at the Olympic Trials Marathon to qualify for the Tokyo Olympics, where she took the bronze medal.

Of course, pro runners aren't any more likely to eat too much than they are to eat too little, and if you want to be the best runner you can be, you'll need to do the same. But how? The task of eating exactly the right amount of calories every single day may seem impossibly daunting, like guessing the number of marbles in a fishbowl or jelly beans in a jar, but it's actually a lot easier than you might assume. Millions of years of evolution went into designing our innate appetite regulatory system, which, under normal circumstances, works beautifully to ensure we eat the right amount. Animals in the wild rely on essentially the same system to control their weight, and when was the last time you saw an overweight or underweight fox in the woods? Human infants are just as good at requesting nourishment when internal signals tell them they need it, and at cutting themselves off when internal signals tell them they've had enough. The only reason so many adults end up overweight in wealthy societies is that environmental factors such as an overabundance of cheap, processed foods and aggressive food marketing train us to override our innate appetite regulatory system and eat when we don't need to.

Going back to eating the right amount of food, as you did naturally when you were a baby, does not require that you calculate your daily calorie needs and rigorously track your calorie intake. Very few professional runners do this with any regularity. What it *does* require is that you base your diet on the types of natural, unprocessed foods our ancestors ate when our innate appetite regulatory system evolved because these foods tend to be far more satiating than modern processed foods, so they fill you up with fewer calories.

This was shown in a study published in *Cell Metabolism* in 2019. Twenty subjects spent four weeks living in a metabolic chamber where their diet could be tightly controlled by researchers. Half the subjects spent the first two weeks on a diet made up of unprocessed (i.e., high-quality) foods and the second two weeks on a diet made up of processed (i.e., low-quality) foods, while the other ten subjects did the opposite. Notably, the two diets contained equal percentages of carbohydrate, fat, and protein, and the subjects were allowed to self-determine the amount of food they ate on both diets. On average, the subjects voluntarily ate 508 fewer calories per day on the unprocessed diet and lost two pounds, whereas they gained two pounds on the processed diet.

173

The second thing you can do to get back to eating the right amount of food is to practice appetite awareness. Whether you are a mindless eater who tends to eat too much or a restrained eater who tends to eat too little, retraining yourself to listen to and heed your body's signals of hunger and satiety will help correct the problem. Here are some basic tips for practicing appetite awareness:

- Except on special occasions, don't start eating a meal or snack until you are experiencing physical hunger cues such as a hollow feeling or rumbling in the stomach.
- On the flip side, don't allow physical hunger cues to persist for very long without addressing them by eating something.
- Stop eating when you feel comfortably satisfied rather than stuffed.
- Avoid automatically finishing the food that's in front of you (especially at restaurants and other places where you don't control how much you're served); also avoid eating something just because it's there.
- Consider downloading an app such as the Am I Hungry? Virtual Coach to assist you in the process of improving your appetite awareness.
- If you have a history of disordered eating, consider hiring a registered dietitian who specializes in this area to help you develop appetite awareness. You'll find it well worth the cost.

The good news for those who tend to overeat is that none of these measures requires you to go hungry. Ask any successful pro runner and they'll tell you they don't deprive themselves. The good news for restrained eaters, meanwhile, is that allowing your appetite to determine how much you eat won't cause you to gain weight even if it does result in your eating more. That's because, as I suggested earlier, chronic undereating slows the body's metabolism, causing it to horde the calories you consume instead of putting them to productive use.

A 2018 study by researchers at the University of Agder and the University of Copenhagen found that endurance athletes who regularly experienced energy deficits during the day (meaning their calorie burning significantly exceeded their calorie intake for two hours or longer) exhibited a suppressed resting metabolic rate even when their twenty-four-hour calorie intake matched their calorie needs. In the same study, higher cortisol levels and lower testosterone levels were observed in those athletes who had the largest within-day energy deficits, an indication that such deficits compromised their ability to recover from and adapt to training.

Scientists refer to this phenomenon as relative energy deficiency in sport (RED-S), and it is as costly as it is common. Just ask Elise Cranny, a member of the Bowerman Track Club who struggled with bone injuries, amenorrhea, and other problems in college as a result of RED-S before rebounding to run 14:48 for 5000 meters and becoming a public advocate for RED-S awareness. "When energy output is greater than energy input," Elise wrote on Instagram in 2020, "both the body and mind can't function at optimal levels. Fueling properly to support training volume and intensity is crucial for mental health, physical health, reproductive health, and overall quality of life."

The lesson from both science and the real world is clear: if you want to run like a pro, you need to eat enough—not just every day but throughout the day!

EAT INDIVIDUALLY

When nonelite runners decide to try to improve their diet, their first move is often to buy a book written by some fad-diet promoter. When elite runners decide to try to improve their diet, their first move is to hire a properly credentialed professional—specifically a registered dietitian or someone with an MS or PhD in nutrition science or exercise physiology. There are two key differences between these professionals and bestsellers written by fad-diet promoters. One is that the professionals don't promote fad diets. The second is that, whereas fad diets offer a plan that's one-size-fits-all, the true experts ask their clients a lot of questions and make a significant effort to tailor solutions to the individual. That's because they understand that each person is metabolically unique, and also that their clients are more likely to sustain improved eating habits if these improvements are limited to necessary changes. Why overhaul when you can simply tweak?

I used to write a column for my Racing Weight blog called "How the Pros Eat." In each installment, I shared details about the diet of an elite endurance athlete. Among those who agreed to share their personal eating habits on this platform were the late Gabriele "Gabe" Grunewald, who was the 2014 US champion at 3000 meters, and 2016 Olympic Triathlon gold medalist turned pro runner Gwen Jorgensen. All of the athletes featured in "Eat Like a Pro" adhered to the four eating habits I've already described, yet no two ate precisely the same. Each had found their own dietary happy place within the parameters defined by the four unbreakable rules of optimal nutrition for endurance fitness and performance. Gwen, for example, told me she preferred to eat hot lunches such as curries, whereas Gabe was more of a sandwich-and-soup type. When I quiz pro runners about why they eat the way they do, they always state specific reasons, which are based on the following six factors: culture, preferences, trial and error, allergies/intolerances, lifestyle, and values.

Culture: It's possible to eat optimally for running within any cultural dietary tradition. If you're Mexican, for example, and you like culturally familiar foods such as tortillas and pinto beans, you do not need to leap over to a Mediterranean diet to become the best runner you can be. Just refine your diet within whichever dietary tradition is familiar and comfortable for you. Even American-style hamburgers can be made with high-quality foods.

Preferences: It is far more likely that you will be successful in sustaining your improved diet over the long term if it is made up of foods you like and if it excludes foods you don't like. There are thousands of different foods to choose from; even the fussiest eater can identify enough foods they enjoy to create a complete, high-quality diet. If there are only four vegetables you like, then eat only those four vegetables—at least to start.

Trial and error: Professional runners tend to be highly attuned to their bodies. This somatic self-awareness leads them to fine-tune their diet over time in ways that make it work better for them. Late in her career, 2018 New York City Marathon winner Shalane Flanagan noticed that she craved sugar during periods of heavy training. On the advice of her nutritionist and friend Elyse Kopecky, Shalane added more high-quality fat-rich foods such as nuts and fish to her diet, and the cravings went away, making it easier for her to attain her optimal racing weight. Whenever you encounter a problem in your running that may have a dietary cause, go through a similar trial-and-error process to identify a possible solution.

Allergies/intolerances: I've mentioned that NAZ Elite member Stephanie Bruce has celiac disease and food allergies. She wasn't always aware of these conditions, however, and they affected her running negatively until testing revealed them, empowering Steph to make the necessary adjustments to her diet. Don't resign yourself to just living with symptoms that hurt your running and could signal a potential food allergy or intolerance. Imagine your livelihood depends on your fitness and performance and do what pros like Steph do in such situations: see a physician.

Lifestyle: Some runners like to cook, others don't. Some have demanding jobs, others don't. Some have children, others don't. But every runner's diet has to conform to their unique lifestyle. As with culture, there is no particular lifestyle that makes it impossible to eat optimally for running. You may just need to accept the realities of your situation—and perhaps get creative. For 2017 US Marathon champion Sara Hall, life got a lot more complicated when she and her husband, Ryan, adopted four girls from Ethiopia. One of the adjustments Sara made was incorporating a lot of teff (the grain used to make injera bread) into the family's diet. Not only did this adjustment make her new daughters happy, but teff is very high in iron and therefore a good thing for any runner to eat.

Values: Jim Walmsley, the elite ultrarunner I mentioned earlier, doesn't eat meat. It's not that he doesn't like meat or that he thinks it's unhealthy. Rather, Jim gave up meat purely for ethical reasons. All the food choices we make have consequences for the world beyond us. It's possible and arguably even important to make choices that support not just your running but also your morals and ethics. If the pros can do it, so can you!

177

Coach's Tip

Food Is Fuel

When I began coaching the NAZ Elite team in January 2014, we had nine athletes. Four of those athletes, now all in their mid-to-late thirties, are still on the team as of this writing, and three of them finished in the top twenty at the 2020 Olympic Trials Marathon. When I was running professionally in the early 2000s, there were hardly any athletes this age still competing at their best. I believe a number of different factors are contributing to the longevity of today's pros, and nutrition is certainly near the top of the list.

All too many professional runners of my generation shared the dietary philosophy of fictional runner Quenton Cassidy, of whom John L. Parker Jr. wrote in the cult classic *Once a Runner*: "He was not a health nut, was not out to mold himself a stylishly slim body. He did not live on nuts and berries; if the furnace was hot enough, anything would burn, even Big Macs." I really wanted to believe these words were true, and if I'm being honest, I still believe they're half true, but half true is also half false. An elite runner who burns five thousand calories a day might be able to get away with a substandard diet for a while, but doing things like running a personal-best marathon time of 2:27:47 in the thirteenth year of one's professional running career, as Stephanie Bruce did in Chicago in 2019, requires aiming for a higher standard. And if *you* also want to run *your* best for as long as possible, and slow down as little as possible as you age, then nutrition should be a key ingredient in your life as well.

Eating like today's professional runners doesn't mean copying exactly what these people eat for breakfast, lunch, and dinner. Instead, it means doing the work that's required to find the best diet and nutrition practices for you. Steph is an especially good role model in this regard because of certain limitations that Matt detailed in chapter 8.

Let's first go all the way back to her collegiate days at the University of California, Santa Barbara. A sub-five-minute-miler in high school, Steph was a top recruit for a program that was good but not great by NCAA Division I standards. She helped change that, eventually leading her cross-country team to a top-ten finish at the NCAA championships in 2006. But it was earlier that same year that she began to understand the correlation between nutrition and performance.

After a great start to the track season that saw her smash her personal best at 10,000 meters and establish herself as one of the best collegiate 10K runners in the country, Steph began to experience extreme fatigue as the national championships approached. With only a couple of weeks until the big day, she finally got some blood work done to see what might be wrong. It turned out that her ferritin level was dangerously low—4 nanograms/milliliter on a scale where normal is between 15 and 150. Ferritin is a blood protein that contains iron, which is an essential component of the process that creates hemoglobin, which in turn is responsible for transporting oxygen in the blood. Low iron levels can result in anemia, in which the body's tissues aren't getting enough oxygen, leaving one feeling weak and tired. A low ferritin level like Steph's indicates that the body is not operating at full oxygen-carrying capacity.

Steph was advised to increase her ferritin levels by taking an iron supplement and to eat iron-rich foods such as red meat. She did so, and by the time the race came around, she was feeling somewhat better. On race day, Steph went deep into the well, leaving everything she had on the track, and she finished eighth—the final All-American spot, and her first such honor. Only afterward did Steph receive the results of a follow-up blood test, which revealed that her ferritin level had indeed risen, but only to 5 nanograms/milliliter. Clearly, Steph's performance on that occasion had more to do with her grit than with the effectiveness of the nutritional solution she'd been given. Subsequently, though, her ferritin level increased much more and she felt and performed even better as a result.

To tell the full story of Steph's nutritional journey from that point forward would require a separate book, and perhaps she'll write it one day, but I am going to jump ahead to the winter of 2019–2020 and the approach she took to nutrition in preparation for the Olympic Trials Marathon. In the three months leading up to the trials, Steph hired a woman named Lottie Bildirici. Known as @runningonveggies on Instagram, Lottie is a renowned advocate for eating clean, plant-based food. A graduate of the Institute for Integrative Nutrition, she has worked with runners for many years, creating recipes and lecturing on using diet as a tool to enhance performance. Steph, due to her celiac disease, had a more obvious need for someone like Lottie than other members of our team, but after seeing the two of them work together and the results their work produced, I have a deeper appreciation for how important nutrition is to performance for every runner.

In nearly all her prior marathons, including the 2019 Chicago Marathon, where she set her personal best, Steph had struggled with her energy and with a variety of gastrointestinal issues. As a consequence, her marathon performances were not on par with her efforts at other distances. And though I believed in Steph as much as anyone, I began to wonder whether she should skip the marathon trials altogether and try to qualify for Tokyo at 10,000 meters instead. Steph, too, realized she had to do something different, or else her dream of becoming an Olympian in the marathon wasn't going to be realistic, and that's where Lottie came in.

Trying to become an Olympian is no easy task. It requires sacrifice, effort, time, focus—and money. While the team and our sponsors pay for many of the things an athlete needs, sometimes athletes have to invest in themselves. For Steph, that meant spending thousands of dollars in the three months before the trials to work with Lottie. It turned out to be money well spent. Together they turned Steph's diet, which for so long had been a disadvantage, into a major advantage. New (and tasty) recipes allowed Steph's body to absorb all the nutrients it needed. Her energy level remained high throughout the entire training segment. Every single Friday, for the final ten weeks before race day, from sunup to sundown, she ate the exact meals she would eat the day before the race. She was a well-oiled machine.

On February 29, 2020, the most important day of Steph's career to that point, she was 100 percent ready. She did not have to worry about low ferritin levels, or what she had eaten the day before, or whether she'd have to go to the bathroom during the race. She could focus solely on performing. And perform she did, finishing in sixth place and missing the team by a mere nineteen seconds. And though she did fall short of her Olympic dream, the fact that she was able to race with all her body and soul, unencumbered by any nutritional limitations, allowed her to walk away completely satisfied. This was one marathon she wouldn't have to look back on wondering, *What if?*

Steph has been gracious enough to share some of the specific dietary measures that she and Lottie implemented to solve her nutrition-related marathon woes. In presenting them here, I don't mean to suggest that if you implement these same measures you will crush your next marathon. As I've tried to convey, no two runners share the same perfect diet. If you want to copy Steph and other pros, don't copy their recipes, copy the rigorous process that enables them to discover the eating habits that work for them.

STEPH'S "GO-TO" FOODS DURING THE TRIALS SEGMENT

Protein Smoothies

Steph would have these twice a day; the first one post-run, within thirty minutes of finishing a workout or run, and the second one at night before bed.

MINT CHOCOLATE CHIP
Rice protein powder
Fresh mint

Cacao nibs

Frozen banana

Almond milk

PUMPKIN PROTEIN PIE

Cup of canned pumpkin

Nutmeg

Cinnamon

Rice protein powder

Almond milk

Maple syrup

Ice

Things she added into her diet

- Veggies at every meal
- Salad before dinner
- Sweet potatoes with almond butter for breakfast
- Protein smoothie before bed
- Brown rice instead of white rice

Things she removed from her diet

- Added sugars from chocolate bars
- Flavored nut butters
- Frequent trips to Five Guys Burgers
- Corn

Timing

- Never went more than three hours without eating
- Fueled her long runs with Skratch Labs sports drinks and energy gels
- Replaced traditional desserts with nutrient-dense snacks

THINK LIKE A PRO

PEOPLE WHO ACHIEVE HIGH levels of success in business, military service, science, and other professional fields tend to possess certain mental skills and traits beyond a natural inclination. To truly excel in these and other fields, research shows, it's not enough to have a knack for business, military service, science, or whatever. One must also be a good decision maker, have solid people skills, be able to regulate emotions effectively, and more.

What about sports, though? When we think about what makes an elite athlete successful, we generally give most, if not all, of the credit to their body and little or none to their mind. I believe this is simply because sports are more obviously physical than other pursuits. The spectacle of, say, a professional basketball player catching an alley-oop pass in midflight and then dunking the ball behind his head blinds us to everything else besides raw physical ability that goes into making such a feat possible.

The reality, however, is that it takes just as much mind power to reach the top in sports as it does in any other pursuit. Recent discoveries in sport and general psychology have greatly increased overall scientific appreciation for the brain's contribution to elite sports performance. In study after study, world-class athletes have been found, as a group, to think differently than athletes at lower tiers of performance. To give just one example, in a series of experiments conducted as part of the PhD thesis she submitted to the Department of Psychology at the University of Westminster, Beth Parkin exposed elite and nonelite athletes to various decision-making tasks under conditions of low and high risk as well as low and high physical pressure, and found that elite athletes tended to make faster and more consistent decisions under physical pressure.

Such findings are consistent with my own personal observations of elite athletes. Whenever someone asks what surprised me the most about the professional runners I trained with as an honorary member of NAZ Elite, I point to my head. Simply put, these young men and women *had their act together*, making good decisions under pressure with striking consistency. I don't mean to suggest that nonelite runners *don't* have their act together, but in my experience there's an unmistakable difference in the psychologies of the two groups, broadly speaking. This disparity is most noticeable in the context of commonly faced challenges such as bad workouts and injuries, which pro runners tend to deal with more effectively than do the rest of us.

The good news is that any runner can get better at dealing with the sport's challenges—I've seen it happen many times, particularly with athletes I coach personally. In this chapter, I will describe how pro runners handle four of the most common challenges and share tips on how to think like a pro when you experience them in your own training and racing. These challenges are how to start (or start over), bad workouts, injuries, and race discomfort.

HOW TO START

Everyone starts at the beginning. No matter how much potential you have as a runner, on your very first day of running, you have not yet realized any of it. You've made zero progress and you have a long way to go to achieve your initial goal, whatever it may be. Things like completing a half marathon or dipping under six minutes for one mile, which many experienced runners achieve routinely, can seem inconceivable to beginners, for whom every step is torture.

For that matter, experienced runners find themselves in pretty much the same position when starting over after an extended break

184

from, or interruption to, their training. Resuming the training process after an injury or illness, or a hiatus caused by family or career obligations, or by a lapse in motivation is like being a beginner all over again. The difference is that, instead of being intimidated by the inconceivability of achieving feats like completing a half marathon or dipping under six minutes for one mile, these more seasoned runners are burdened by unfavorable comparisons to the runner they were previously. Do any of the following sentiments sound familiar?

"I can't believe how hard nine-minute miles feel now."

"I used to do this workout so much faster."

"Six months ago, I could have climbed that hill in my sleep."

Professional runners sometimes find themselves back at the beginning too, but they are less prone to fretting about how far they have to go to get where they want to be or about how much fitter and faster they were before. As to *how* they steer clear of such self-created psychological traps, it is mainly by maintaining a *process focus* rather than an *outcome focus*. Instead of brooding about where they are in their fitness relative to where they once were or where they want to be, they keep their attention focused on getting fitter.

In 2020, Olympic 800-meter runner Kate Grace suffered an Achilles tendon injury that forced her to take ten weeks off from running, which caused her to lose a lot of fitness. In the early stages of her return to training, when her workout times were far below her prior standards, Kate focused on her effort instead of her splits, drawing confidence from knowing that, numbers notwithstanding, she was at least working as hard as she had before.

Process-focused runners like Kate care just as much about achieving goals as outcome-focused runners do, but they concentrate their attention on *now*, whereas outcome-focused runners give more attention to the future. There's been a lot of research showing that a process focus tends to yield greater improvement in a wide range of pursuits, including sports, so it's not surprising that elite runners strive to maintain this type of focus.

A good example is Ed Eyestone, who won the 1984 NCAA cross country championship as a student at Brigham Young University and then returned to the school in 2000 to coach cross country and track.

By that time, BYU had fallen far from its glory days, but Eyestone had ambitions of bringing the Cougars back to the top. In other words, the program was starting over, as all runners do at one time or another. Eyestone was undeterred, however, because he understood the value and power of being process focused.

One of the things that makes running competitively at BYU more challenging than doing so at other colleges and universities is that most of the student-athletes there take a two-year break from school to serve missions in other countries, where they do not run. Eyestone had done it himself, and he saw this apparent disadvantage as an opportunity to instill a process focus in his runners. Student-athletes returning to campus from mission service are truly back at square one, and therein lies the opportunity. "A seventy-mile-per-week-kid can't just do seventy miles again," Eyestone told *PodiumRunner*'s Johanna Gretschel in a 2020 interview. To keep their minds off this number, Eyestone gives them bite-size goals to work on, the first of which, in most cases, is to jog three miles and report back on how it feels.

Even when runners have come all the way back, Eyestone keeps them process focused. The BYU men's cross country team came into the 2019 NCAA championship as a contender to win, having placed second the year before. And their goal was indeed to win, but that's not what Eyestone had his runners focus on. Instead, he gave each member of the team a concrete plan for "winning" his individual race—meaning not necessarily to cross the finish line first but to execute the best race possible. "We were focused on doing our best because we knew we could do our best and win it, or we could do our best and take third," Cougar senior Conner Mantz told *Daily Herald* reporter Jared Lloyd after the race. "We weren't focusing so much on the result but instead we were focusing on the process." As it turned out, doing their best *did* result in victory for Conner and his teammates.

It's one thing to buy into the idea of maintaining a process focus, another thing to actually do it. One very simple yet powerful way to develop and maintain a process focus is to set and pursue process goals, much as Ed Eyestone does with his BYU runners returning from missionary work. There's nothing wrong with having big outcome goals such as lowering your 10K personal best or completing your first 50K trail race, but achieving such goals will be all the more likely if you use process goals as stepping-stones along the way. Examples of process goals are keeping your heart rate below 140 beats per minute throughout all your easy runs; finding time for drills twice a week every week, no excuses; increasing your average weekly mileage by 10 percent in your next training cycle; and squeezing in at least one trail run per week.

Another simple tool you can use to maintain a process focus is self-talk. I like to give runners mantras to recite internally before, during, and after runs to encourage a process focus. One of my favorites, which I picked up from Coach Ben, is "Get better today." This concise self-command serves as a helpful reminder that it doesn't matter how fit you are today in relation to your past peaks or your future ambitions. What matters is whether you're getting fitter, and if you are executing a sensible training plan step-by-step, you are getting a little better each day.

Another mantra you can use to the same effect is "Check the box." Not every run can be, or needs to be, a huge breakthrough. Even the most successful training cycles—ones that culminate in Olympic medals and national records—are made up mostly of check-the-box type runs. I encourage you to use mantras like these to keep your mind on *now* as you make your way through the training process.

BAD WORKOUTS

One of the most important functions of the training process is to build confidence. Rarely do runners achieve race goals they aren't confident they can achieve when they step up to the start line. In addition to developing the fitness runners need to achieve their goals, training must also supply them with proof they're on track to succeed. No matter how well the training process goes, however, it never goes so well that *every* important workout builds confidence. Bad workouts are inevitable. With good planning and proper execution, these disappointments can be kept to a minimum, but no runner ever gets through a full training cycle without bombing once or twice.

In my experience, pro runners generally deal with bad workouts more skillfully than nonelite runners do. The difference lies in how much significance each group gives to training sessions that don't go well. Nonelite runners tend to put a lot of weight on them, seeing them as evidence of low fitness or even lack of running ability. Pro runners place less significance on bad workouts, dismissing them as a consequence of fatigue or as "just one of those days" or even interpreting them positively as proof that they're really working hard in their training—paying dues that will be rewarded in time.

The upshot of these contrasting responses to bad workouts is that pro runners gain more confidence from their training than the rest of us do. Elites and nonelites alike get a confidence boost from good workouts, whereas only nonelites (with plenty of exceptions, of course) lose confidence in the wake of a bad workout. Picture two runners standing at the start of an important race, both of whom experienced eleven good workouts and three bad workouts in the lead-up to the event. Which of these runners is more likely to achieve their goal: the one who shook off those bad workouts or the one who took them to heart? The answer is obvious.

The pros aren't only wise but also *right* to dismiss bad workouts as being not truly indicative of their fitness level. Although bad workouts are sometimes evidence of an underlying problem such as a nutrient deficiency or inadequate recovery, bad workouts of the more common, inevitable kind really aren't reliable indicators of fitness. Think about it: No runner can possibly perform beyond their physical capacity in a workout. If you do something in a workout, it's because you are fit enough to do it, period. There are no miracles or flukes.

Bad workouts are a different story. It's quite easy to perform below the level of your fitness in a given workout due to preexisting fatigue or any number of other factors, such as mental exhaustion from a tough day at the office, that are bound to crop up in the course of training. It is simply *reasonable*, therefore, to look to your better training sessions for evidence of your current fitness level and to dismiss your less successful runs for what they typically are: negative exceptions to a positive trend. And by the same token, it's unreasonable to allow a single subpar run to lower your confidence level. If a bad workout does impact your confidence, the problem isn't the workout, it's your confidence.

Toward the end of my summer with NAZ Elite, the team did a long run in which, for whatever reason, almost everyone felt lousy and performed poorly. Afterward I listened with keen interest as the runners conducted a kind of verbal postmortem. It was instructive to hear how those who'd laid an egg that morning talked through their disappointment and how those who'd run well helped them in this process.

"I've never had a marathon segment where I didn't have at least one terrible workout," said Sarah Crouch, an independent pro who sometimes ran with the team. "No matter how well the segment as a whole is going, it always happens."

"It's one workout," said Matt Llano, one of the few runners who'd actually run well that morning. "You can't put too much on it. You already know you're fit—you've proven that a thousand times in the past several weeks. Days like these are bound to happen and they shouldn't rattle you."

I came away from the experience with a renewed appreciation for how helpful it is to process bad workouts verbally. Here again, what works for the elites can work for you, too. If you're a runner who struggles to shake off bad workouts, get in the habit of talking them through with a coach or fellow runner. The simple act of putting the experience into words will help you gain perspective on it, and your chosen sounding board can help you further by chiming in from a more objective angle. In some cases, it will be possible to identify an obvious reason for your underperformance, be it unfavorable weather or tired legs or a dip in motivation or something else. Other times there will be no clear culprit and you and your sounding board will need to do what Sarah and Matt did, which is to write off the workout as a normal, if unpleasant, part of the training experience.

An alternative to a human sounding board is a journal or log. Cat Bradley, a professional ultrarunner whom I happen to coach, keeps a daily journal that she uses to record both the good and the bad in her running journey. Other runners use their training log to gain perspective on their worries, or share them with a Facebook running

189

group. And, speaking of training logs, one other measure that I find helpful after a bad workout is to review my most recent *good* workout in my training log as a way to remind myself how fit I really am.

INJURIES

The wisest words that have ever been spoken on the topic of running injuries, in my humble opinion, were spoken by 2:12 marathoner Jason Lehmkuhle in a 2009 interview. "I think that you just have to accept that you are probably going to get injured every once in a while," he said. "It's part of the sport. The way that you *deal* with the injury is probably more important than trying to do everything to prevent injuries."

I couldn't agree more. Every runner shares the goal of minimizing the degree to which injuries disrupt their training and racing, and the runners who deal with injuries the most skillfully are the least affected by them. Psychologists favor the term *coping* over the less formal *dealing with* when discussing how people think about the challenges they face. Successful injury coping is all about managing emotions constructively and exercising good judgment, and professional runners tend to do both.

A case in point is an interaction I had with NAZ Elite runner Aaron Braun one Sunday. We had both just completed depletion runs—twenty-two miles for me and twenty-six miles for him—and when I asked Aaron how his run had gone, he told me he'd bailed out a couple of miles early because a hip injury he'd been training through was bothering him.

"That's too bad," I said reflexively.

"Not really," he said. "I could have pushed through it and finished, but why risk it? I'd rather miss out on a couple of miles today and be able to train one hundred percent next week than force those two miles and pay for it."

I'm sure this reasoning sounds as sensible to you as it did to me in the moment, but how many other runners would have made the same sensible decision in Aaron's place? I can say with confidence that very few of the runners I've ever coached would have done so. Instead,

190

driven by fear of missing out on the benefits of those last two miles, or anticipating the sense of failure they'd be saddled with if they didn't complete the prescribed distance, most would have rolled the dice and gone the full twenty-six—and regretted it later, in all likelihood. In other words, they would have allowed emotion rather than reason to govern their decision.

Emotions aren't bad; they exist for a purpose. But intense emotions have a way of clouding our judgment and causing us to make poor decisions. Because injuries threaten something that is precious to us, they churn up strong emotions—fear, anxiety, frustration, anger, and grief—that result in boneheaded choices, which in turn make avoidable injuries inevitable and needlessly prolong existing injuries, while also making the injury experience more unpleasant than it needs to be. Imagine Mr. Spock, the impassive half-Vulcan character from the old TV series *Star Trek*, as a runner. We can assume the pointy-eared space traveler would take a coldly rational problem-solving approach to making decisions around injuries. This is pretty much what professional runners must do.

I'm reminded of a comment Coach Ben made on Instagram in 2018 about Stephanie Bruce, who had just finished second in the US Marathon Championship with a personal-best time of 2:29:21 (since lowered), an accomplishment that was all the more impressive having come only weeks after a disappointing performance at the New York City Marathon. "My initial reaction was that she was thinking emotionally, rather than rationally," Ben wrote concerning Steph's post-NYC appeal to let her jump into the unplanned second marathon. "She assured me that was not the case, however, and laid out her reasoning in a very calm manner." Specifically, Steph persuaded Ben that there was no harm in trying because she could always bail out of the training or the race itself if her body wasn't up to it and she had no other races planned until the following year, for which she would have plenty of time to recover regardless.

This example nicely illustrates how, even when strong emotions such as disappointment drive pro runners to flout conventional practices (very seldom do sponsored runners contest two marathons in the span of a month) and take calculated risks, they and their coaches

191

remain on guard against allowing those emotions to rule the decision-making process. Admittedly, avoiding irrational, emotion-based decisions as a runner is easier if, like Steph, you have a coach.

If you're self-coached, making good decisions will require that you cultivate your inner Spock—an internal voice of reason that plays the same role a coach would play on your behalf if you had one. This works best if, when you step into your Spock role, you regard your athletic self as a separate person, someone whose best interests you have at heart. When I perform this exercise, I sometimes pretend my athlete self is a character in a book I'm reading, a protagonist I'm rooting for but with a degree of detachment.

Admittedly, it's not quite as easy as it sounds. Achieving the same level of judgment the pros have will require that you train yourself to take a mental step back from your situation each and every time you face a decision that has implications for injury avoidance or injury management (e.g., "Should I rest this sore foot or go ahead with to-day's scheduled run?"). You'll have to do this again and again before it becomes instinctual and you're consistently able to make decisions that subjugate emotion to reason, but you won't regret the effort.

Woven into the fabric of most injury-related decisions is uncertainty. Much of the anxiety runners feel around injury is rooted in the lack of answers. But not all runners are equally troubled by uncertainty, and those who are least troubled by it tend to make the best injury-related decisions. Professional runners have a way of arriving at a wise acceptance of the uncertainty surrounding injuries. As Jason Lehmkuhle put it, "It has certainly been my experience that if you try to figure it out, you will just drive yourself crazy." His point here is not that runners should make no effort whatsoever to identify and address the causes of injuries, but that runners should not make the mistake of assuming they have to have perfect information to manage injuries effectively. Pro runners focus on controlling the controllable and accepting the uncontrollable as just that, and you should do the same.

RACE DISCOMFORT

If my favorite quote about running injuries comes from Jason Lehmkuhle, my favorite quote about the suffering that runners experience during races (and hard workouts) is from legendary ultrarunner Scott Jurek: "Pain only hurts." In other words, as intense as it may be, the discomfort we experience when running to our limit does no harm beyond being uncomfortable. Sure, it might feel like you're dying, but you're not. Some runners, including the pros (who wouldn't be pros otherwise), have a higher tolerance for this sort of discomfort than others do. Those who maintain a pain-only-hurts attitude toward their suffering have the highest tolerance for it and consequently get the most out of the physical fitness they bring to each race.

What does it mean, though, to have a pain-only-hurts attitude? At its core, it's about not making race discomfort out to be more than it really is. To say that pain only hurts is to accept the pain as a necessary part of the racing experience instead of wishing it away as though it were an indication that something has gone wrong. Former 5000 meter American record holder Bob Kennedy said it well: "One thing about racing is that it hurts. You better accept that from the beginning or you're not going anywhere."

Accepting discomfort does not lessen it, but it does make it more tolerable, hence less of a drag on performance. Research has shown that people who are trained to accept exercise-related discomfort experience lower perceived effort levels and perform better in endurance tests. A 2011 study by scientists at the Catholic University of America, for example, found that high school runners trained in mindfulness techniques (a practice that involves acceptance of internal states and external circumstances) significantly lowered their mile times.

Two good ways to increase your acceptance of race discomfort are *bracing* and *detachment*. Bracing entails actively girding your mind for suffering before a race. Tell yourself, *This is going to hurt*, and be okay with that. Never allow yourself to be unpleasantly surprised by how much you hurt during competition. Detachment entails separating your thoughts and emotions from your perceptions so that the latter don't control the former. Realize that you don't have to think negative thoughts and experience unpleasant emotions just because your esophagus is on fire and your legs feel like concrete. Instead of thinking *I hate this* at such moments, think *I've been here before and gotten through it. This is nothing new.*

Psychologists refer to this type of process as *metacognition*, which can be loosely defined as thinking about your thoughts and feelings. The better you are at observing your own consciousness, the more you can control it. It should come as no surprise to learn that elite runners rely heavily on metacognition when racing. In 2015, sports psychologist Noel Brick of Ulster University teamed up with a pair of colleagues to interview ten elite runners about what went on in their heads during competition. A majority of these athletes described not merely feeling intense discomfort in races but also using the sensation as information. In a discussion of their findings published in *Psychology of Sport and Exercise,* Brick and his coauthors remarked, "While many athletes reported awareness of exertional pain during running, this awareness was primarily used as a signal to engage an appropriate cognitive strategy." In essence, the runners asked themselves, "Given how I'm feeling right now, what is the best thought I can think or the best action I can take to maximize my performance?" Among the most commonly cited responses to discomfort were adjusting pace, trying to relax, and "chunking" distance or time (i.e., mentally dividing a run into smaller segments to make the distance seem more manageable).

The researchers noted that while certain specific metacognitive strategies were widely practiced among these elite runners, others were idiosyncratic. What matters most is not the specific thing you think or do in response to discomfort but that you cultivate a habit of monitoring (rather than just feeling) your discomfort so you can choose the best response *for you.* As a coach, I've found that different metacognitive strategies are useful to different athletes. When I find myself deep in the pain cave in races, my self-talk becomes rather harsh ("Man up! Don't be a wimp!"). It works for me, but when I share this strategy with my athletes, some of them look at me like I need to be locked up.

In fact, though, my little mid-race drill-sergeant routine is nothing more than an idiosyncratic way of exercising what's known as *inhibitory control*, which all runners exercise in one way or another. Inhibitory control is the ability to resist immediate impulses (such as the desire to slow down or quit for the sake of escaping discomfort) and stay focused on a less immediate goal (such as completing a race in the least time possible). The better you get at vetoing your urges to take your foot off the gas in races, the better you will perform. In a 2015 study, Italian researchers found that a standard test of inhibitory control was a strong predictor of subsequent race performance in a group of ultrarunners.

Other research has shown that inhibitory control can be strengthened through deliberate practice, and there are lots of ways to do this. In everyday life, just about any form of deferred gratification you can think of will strengthen the underlying mechanism, which is centered in a part of the brain called the anterior cingulate cortex. An example from my own life is creating a daily to-do list and tackling the item I dread most first, the item I'm most looking forward to last. In training, things like exercising to failure (e.g., holding a wall squat as long as you can) and the aforementioned mental trick of chunking distance or time when you're running hard will have the same effect.

Metacognition is also useful for emotional self-regulation. Individuals who are adept at regulating their emotions are said to have a high level of emotional intelligence (EI), and guess what: Research has shown that EI, too, correlates with running performance. A study led by Enrico Rubaltelli of the University of Padova and published in *Personality and Individual Differences* in 2018 found that individual scores on a test of EI predicted half-marathon performance better than prior racing experience and even training volume in a group of recreational runners.

Emotional intelligence, too, can be increased through deliberate practice. Mindfulness training is one proven means of enhancing the capacity for emotional self-regulation. But there are other ways. A lot of runners, including many professionals, use the training and racing context itself to work on this skill. Simply recognizing that you always have a degree of freedom to choose your emotions is half the

195

battle; from this point, it is relatively easy to choose specific emotions that are more helpful than reflexive fear. If your shoe spontaneously falls apart during a marathon, for instance (as happened to Eliud Kipchoge during the 2015 Berlin Marathon), you don't have to panic; you can keep calm and press on (as Eliud did, ultimately winning the race).

You may find it easier to control your emotions during a race if you preselect a desired emotional state before it even starts. Some elite runners like to race angry, and intentionally work themselves into a lather prior to competing. There is scientific evidence that anger can indeed be performance-enhancing for certain runners. Others have had success racing in a state of gratitude, especially when returning from a setback. Ryan Hall made a conscious choice to race the 2010 Boston Marathon with joy, and it helped him achieve a fourth-place, 2:08:40 performance. The fact that the fastest American-born marathoner in history chose to race happy is all the proof we need that having fun and performing at the highest level are not mutually incompatible.

The Champion's Mind-Set

It is my belief, having coached elite athletes for many years, that the mind is the great separator between the very good and the truly great. In a book I wrote with my high school coach Jim Linhares about building a high school cross country program, we refer to the mental makeup of the truly great as a champion's mind-set. Now, as a professional coach who has to make decisions about which athletes to add to our roster, I am only interested in those who possess this mind-set.

I have been fortunate to find many such athletes in the past several years, and I could certainly use any number of them as examples in this chapter. But the first runner who comes to mind is a guy who might well be the fiercest competitor, intrinsically, I have ever known: Scott Fauble. And I say *intrinsically* because, in running, most of the battles we fight are in our own mind. As Matt mentions, we have to cope, or deal, with injuries. We have to analyze bad workouts in a pragmatic way. And above all, if we want to perform to the absolute best of our ability, we have to embrace the inescapable discomfort that comes from pushing one's body to the limit. Scott Fauble embraces this discomfort as well as or better than anyone I have ever known.

But it wasn't always that way. Matt makes the point that we can all get better at dealing with the sport's challenges, and Scott has certainly done so. A high school state champion and national finalist in cross country, Scott was blessed with blue-chip talent. He chose to run collegiately at the University of Portland, a small school but one with a decades-long tradition of producing great distance runners. But just as there are difficult decisions to make in races, there are difficult decisions to make in college. As Scott would tell you, he made some poor decisions his freshman year. Those decisions—most notably choosing partying over sleep—led to many a subpar performance on the cross-country course and on the track. But champions learn from their mistakes. By his sophomore year, Scott was making the right decisions and never again ran poorly in cross-country, improving from twenty-sixth to thirteenth to twelfth at the NCAA cross country championships in 2012, 2013, and 2014.

With his mind-set headed in the right direction, Scott made the leap to professional running in the summer of 2015, when he signed with our team. He did so, however, coming off the first major injury of his career—a metatarsal stress fracture. In fact, when he made his recruiting trip to Flagstaff, he was in a boot. Remember what Matt told you: as a runner, you are probably going to get injured at some point. For Scott, in retrospect, I believe this may have been a blessing in disguise. It forced him as a rookie to deal with some adversity, something that will inevitably be a part of any athlete's career eventually. He coped with that stress fracture like a champion. Instead of sulking and wallowing in self-pity, he got in the pool and aqua-jogged, he worked on his core, and when it was time to come back to running, he did so cautiously, believing that he'd be better than ever soon enough, and indeed he was.

Of course, many pros partied too much in their first year of college, and I know firsthand that nearly all of them have handled injuries in a smart way. What sets Scott apart from his peers is his ability to go deeper into the well in the toughest moments of a race than many have ever dared to go. I'll use the 2019 Boston Marathon as an example. Boston was Scott's third marathon. He had made his debut in the fall of 2017 in Frankfurt, Germany, where he'd run 2:12:35. A year later, he ran 2:12:28 on the difficult New York City course, finishing in seventh place. So he was certainly off to a great start, but not necessarily someone you'd expect to be contending for the win up against many of the world's best marathoners in Boston.

Nevertheless, I can assure you that Scott walked up to that starting line in Hopkinton as confident as any runner in the field. His training had been phenomenal. He had done things he'd never done before, things no one on our team had ever done, things that told us unequivocally he was in great shape. Still, being seeded twenty-seventh out of the twenty-nine elite men in the race would cause many a runner to question whether they truly belonged, regardless of how fit they were. But remember, running is largely an interior battle. As a runner, you don't have to allow your circumstances to rule your thoughts and emotions. You don't have to react to a daunting challenge by running scared. You can instead, if you so dare, take a huge risk not really knowing what's going to happen, living only in the present moment, which is precisely what Scott Fauble did in the 2019 Boston Marathon.

In the first half of the race, Scott ran in what I would describe as a very free, yet calculated, way. He settled into a rhythm that seemed comfortable internally, not concerned with anything going on around him, not caring exactly what pace he was running, going entirely by feel. That rhythm, which was about 4:55 per mile, put him near the front much of the time. But around twelve miles, fellow American Jared Ward broke the race open with an aggressive surge that Scott chose not to go with. His quick mental calculations told him it wasn't right, even though physically he could have done it. At halfway, he had fallen thirteen seconds behind the leaders and into twentieth place. From mile fifteen to mile sixteen, however, the course drops one hundred feet. Having done a ton of downhill work in practice, Scott felt comfortable on the descent and let his legs go, running that mile in 4:35 and making his way all the way back to the head of the race.

Then the real racing began. The famous Newton Hills were upon them, and they wouldn't relent until the twenty-one-mile mark. And it was there, in the toughest part of the race, that Scott threw calculations out the window and began racing in the moment. Between 25K and 30K he moved from sixteenth place to first. Yes, Scott Fauble was leading the Boston Marathon 18.6 miles into the race!

199

At twenty miles, at the base of Heartbreak Hill, the lead pack had been whittled down to just eleven men—and Scott had done most of the whittling. By twenty-one miles, only eight runners were left in contention, the last big climb having taken three more victims. At this point, with five miles to go, most runners with Scott's credentials would simply be thanking their lucky stars they had made it this far, perhaps thinking, *Hey, if I can just run decently over this last bit I'll make the top ten.* When I spoke to Scott afterward, though, he told me something I will never forget. With five miles remaining in the race, up against athletes with personal bests more than eight minutes faster than his own, he thought, *I know I can crush these last four miles. Maybe if I go hard enough, I can get away and win.*

And crush them he did. Scott covered the distance between the 35K and 40K marks of the race in 15:04—his fastest 5K split of the day. Unfortunately, it wasn't enough. Scott finished seventh in 2:09:09, but his time was a personal best by more than three minutes and made him the eleventh-fastest American marathoner of all time.

Matt mentioned that he likes to give his athletes mantras to use in races, so I will leave you with a famous Scott Fauble mantra, one that he has used many times, including with one mile to go at Boston, when he was in more pain than he'd ever been in at any point in any race he'd ever run: "You can go deeper, Scott. You can take more." Here's an idea: The next time you race, substitute Scott's name with yours and see if this mantra doesn't help you, too, compete like a champion.

TRAINING PLANS OVERVIEW

THE FIVE CHAPTERS THAT follow this overview offer a collection of fifteen training plans targeting five popular race distances: 5K, 10K, half marathon, marathon, and ultramarathon. There are three plans for each distance, organized by level. The level 1 plans are designed for less experienced runners and for runners who either need or prefer a lower-volume program. The level 2 plans are suited for runners with a training background that is sufficient to allow them to handle a moderately high workload. The level 3 plans feature a heavy workload that closely matches that of professional runners.

All the plans are built on the principles and methods by which the pros train but are not derived from any specific athlete or team. It's unlikely you will find one that is a perfect match for you exactly as it's written. For example, each plan builds up to a single race at the end, but you may wish to do one or more other races in the lead-up to that event, in which case some adjustments will be necessary. I'm confident the things you've learned in reading the preceding chapters will enable you to make sensible adjustments fairly easily.

One thing you may notice in perusing the plans is that they are fairly similar across race distances. This is because, as both Coach Ben and I have noted, the pros train similarly for races of different distances. Among the more common training mistakes that nonelite runners make is over-specializing in their race preparations. Those aiming at shorter events such as 5Ks tend to do a lot of speed work and not a lot of volume or long running, while those preparing for longer events such as marathons tend to do the opposite. In contrast, the pros train at high volume, maintain an approximate 80/20 intensity balance, and draw from the same set of tried-and-true workout formats regardless of the distance of their next event. Remember what Stephanie Bruce said to Coach Ben after winning a half marathon and setting a 5K personal best in the span of eleven days on the same training? "When you're fit, you're fit!"

All fifteen training plans feature three-week step cycles, with a recovery week scheduled every third week. In the level 2 and level 3 plans, these weeks begin with a rest day. In the level 1 plans, which include a rest day every week, it is an overall reduction in running that makes recovery weeks easier than the preceding weeks of the step cycle.

Certain terminology used in the plans requires a bit of decoding. The following table does this. Refer back to it as often as necessary as you make your way through your chosen plan. Note that there are a few workouts scattered throughout the plans that key off one of these intensities without directly targeting it. For example, a particular workout might have you run a segment at lactate-threshold pace plus five seconds per mile.

As described in chapter 4, a shading system is used to distinguish runs of different challenge levels. Runs expected to be highly challenging are designated by dark shading, moderately challenging runs are marked by light shading, and easy runs appear in unshaded boxes. Don't make too much of these designations, though. For example, in certain plans, long runs scheduled in the early weeks are designated as unchallenging, while the bigger long runs scheduled in later weeks are designated as moderately or highly challenging, based on the expectation that, for most runners, the long runs will get harder as they get longer. But it's possible that you will find the long runs in a given plan somewhat hard from the beginning, or that they won't become challenging for you until faster segments are incorporated into them. Neither scenario is bad as long as you aren't completely overwhelmed by the runs.

There are eighteen different run types represented in the plans. Here are a few guidelines on how to execute them.

INTENSITY	MEANING
Easy	At or below your VT_1 pace, heart rate, or power (see chapter 4 for guidelines on determining these values)
Marathon Pace (MP)	Your current or goal marathon race pace
Steady-State Pace (SSP)	The fastest pace you could sustain for two hours
Half-Marathon Pace (MP)	Your current or goal half-marathon race pace
Lactate-Threshold Pace (LTP)	The fastest pace you could sustain for one hour
10K Pace (10KP)	Your current or goal 10K race pace
Critical Velocity (CV)	The fastest pace you could sustain for thirty minutes
High Intensity (HI)	The range between critical velocity and maximum aerobic speed
5K Pace (5KP)	Your current or goal 5K race pace
Maximum Aerobic Speed (MAS)	The fastest pace you could sustain for six minutes
Very-High Intensity (VHI)	The range between maximum aerobic speed and a full sprint

EASY RUNS

Execute these runs according to the guidelines presented in chapter 5. Above all, remember that if you can't speak comfortably in complete sentences, you're running too fast, and that you should let your pace fluctuate between, and even within, easy runs based on how you feel, never allowing your perceived effort level to exceed 4 out of 10.

LONG RUNS

Long runs take various forms, the most basic of which is simply an easy run that lasts longer than most easy runs do. No matter where you place it, the dividing line between easy runs and long runs is arbitrary. Is a seventy-minute run at low intensity a longish easy run or a shorter long run? It doesn't really matter. Regardless of what you call it, you're running for seventy minutes at low intensity.

You'll find that some plans feature duration-based long runs and others distance-based long runs. Duration-based long runs are generally preferable, as they ensure that runners of all abilities get an equivalent training stimulus. A fifteen-mile run, for example, is a bigger test for a slower runner who needs two and a half hours to complete the distance than it is for a faster runner who can bang it out in one hour and forty-five minutes. But the reality is that a marathon is indeed a longer race for slower runners than it is for faster runners, so the plans I've built for this distance feature distance-based long runs to ensure that slower runners are no less prepared to go the full distance.

Training plans for even longer events—ultramarathons—feature duration-based runs. This may seem to contradict the principle I just articulated, and in a sense it does, but with good reason. Most ultramarathons take more than five hours for even the swiftest runners to complete, yet no runner is capable of gaining fitness from a training run lasting longer than five hours. Anything longer isn't training—it's punishment. Hence, it's best to do duration-based long runs in ultra training and to cap them at five hours.

In addition to basic long runs, which serve to develop the raw endurance needed to cover a given race distance, there are a variety of fancier long-run types sprinkled among many of the training plans. Depletion runs (described in chapter 8) are long runs completed without calorie intake before or during their execution. Long runs with surges, long runs with tempo, long fast-finish runs, and long progression runs all include bouts of faster running that impose an additional fitness-boosting challenge beyond that of merely completing a given duration or distance. Each in its own way teaches the body to run fast in a fatigued state.

FAST-FINISH RUNS

Fast-finish runs are used mainly to supply a small dose of moderate-intensity running. You'll find them most often in the early weeks of training and in recovery weeks. The first and longest segment of each fast-finish run is done at low intensity; hence, you should follow my pacing guidelines for easy runs in this part. The fast finish usually targets either lactate-threshold pace or critical velocity.

If, like most runners, you enjoy running fast, think of the fast finish as a reward for holding yourself back during the easy part of the run—the running equivalent of a bowl of ice cream you earn by eating your vegetables.

PROGRESSION RUNS

A progression run is a fast-finish run where the fast part is divided into two or three steps. For example, a given progression run might ask you to run easy for forty minutes, then at lactate-threshold pace for eight minutes, critical velocity for four minutes, and lastly maximum aerobic speed for two minutes. Generally speaking, progression runs are slightly more challenging than fast-finish runs but still less challenging than workouts such as tempo runs that target a moderate intensity.

FARTLEK RUNS

A fartlek run is essentially a casual interval run. Like interval runs, fartleks include fast running, just not as much of it. Fartleks are also like fast-finish runs and progression runs in the sense that they are intended to supply a lighter dose of harder work and are most often scheduled in the early base-building period of training and in recovery weeks.

HILL-REPETITIONS RUNS

Hill repetitions are a sort of cross between speed work and strength training. Similar to high-intensity interval runs, they feature alternating segments of hard and easy running, but because the hard efforts are done uphill, they subject the legs to more of a strength/power challenge. Shorter hill reps target very-high intensity (VHI), while longer hill reps target high intensity (HI). The general idea with hill repetitions is to finish them feeling you put in a 9-out-of-10 effort overall, as described in chapter 5.

TEMPO RUNS

A tempo run is a run that features one or more prolonged efforts at moderate intensity. All the tempo runs included in these fifteen training plans specifically target lactate-threshold pace. Training at this pace will make you more comfortable and efficient at moderate running speeds.

OVER/UNDER INTERVALS RUNS

Over/under intervals are intervals in which the pace fluctuates between slightly above and slightly below lactate-threshold pace. The benefits are more or less the same as those of a tempo run, but the variable-pace format carries the additional benefit of teaching the body to recover from a harder effort while still running somewhat aggressively, and many runners find the frequent pace changes more stimulating than locking into lactate-threshold pace.

STEADY-STATE RUNS

A steady-state run features an extended bout at steady state pace (SSP). These workouts play a vital role in training for longer races, where the goal for many runners is not merely to go the distance but to do so at a fairly aggressive pace.

CRITICAL-VELOCITY RUNS

A critical-velocity run is an interval run in which the fast efforts target critical velocity. These runs serve to increase the speed at which your body can maintain a stable physiological state, thereby delaying exhaustion.

VARIABLE-SPEED INTERVAL RUNS

A variable-speed interval run is a newer type of workout developed by European scientists in which each high-intensity effort toggles between lactate-threshold pace and maximum aerobic speed. Research has shown that this format enables athletes to spend more time above 90 percent of VO_2max within the session, amplifying its fitness-boosting effect.

ACCELERATION RUNS

Conceived by French exercise physiologist Véronique Billat, an acceleration run is a long, gradual acceleration from an easy jog to an all-out sprint. Described in chapter 5, this workout offers a unique physical challenge along with valuable pacing practice.

VO_2MAX RUNS

The plans that follow this overview include a variety of workout formats that target maximum aerobic speed and serve to increase aerobic capacity and improve fatigue resistance at faster running speeds. These include descending interval runs, lactate interval runs, and certain fartlek, fast-finish, and progression runs.

LEG-SPEED RUNS

A leg-speed run is a workout featuring intervals performed at very high intensity. Some leg speed runs call for passive rest between sprints, others for a walk-to-jog recovery, where you begin the recovery period at a walk and transition to easy running when you feel ready. Shorter sprints should be done as nearly all-out efforts, longer ones a bit slower. In either case, focus on staying relaxed and aim to complete the last sprint feeling as though you could do one or two more at the same speed.

5K PACE RUNS

As the name indicates, a 5K pace run is a run that targets 5K race pace (5KP). When a 5K pace run appears in a 5K training plan, the intervals should be run specifically at your 5K goal pace, even if it's a

207

little faster than the pace you could sustain for this distance currently. When a workout of this type appears in a plan focused on a different race distance, run the intervals at your current estimated 5K race pace. This type of workout is always distance-based instead of duration-based because, whether your goal pace is five minutes per mile or ten minutes per mile, you need to be able to sustain it for a full five kilometers.

10K PACE RUNS

A 10K pace run targets 10K race pace (10KP). All of the above guidelines for 5K pace runs apply to 10K pace runs as well.

HALF-MARATHON PACE RUNS

A half-marathon pace run targets half-marathon race pace (HMP). All of the guidelines for 5K pace runs apply to half-marathon pace runs as well.

MARATHON-PACE RUNS

A marathon-pace run targets marathon race pace (MP). All of the guidelines given for 5K pace runs apply to marathon-pace runs as well.

DRILLS, STRIDES, AND PLYOS

Drills and strides are included in the warm-up for faster workouts in all of the training plans. The level 2 plans also prescribe drills and strides after one easy run per week, and the level 3 plans add plyometrics, or plyos. Refer back to chapter 6 for suggested drills and plyos, or feel free to select your own. Strides are fifteen-second relaxed sprints followed by thirty-second passive recoveries. Complete two to four of these before starting the next part of the workout.

CROSS-TRAINING

The level 1 plans give you the option to replace some easy runs with a cross-training session. You may do so either routinely or as needed. The best cross-training activities for runners are those that, like running itself, involve independent leg movements. Examples are indoor and outdoor bicycling, indoor elliptical running, outdoor elliptical biking, and uphill treadmill walking. Although the level 2 and level 3 plans do not explicitly offer a cross-training option, you should feel free also to replace any easy run with a cross-training session in the process of following any of these plans, particularly on days when soreness from prior running makes high-impact activity seem inadvisable.

COACH BEN'S FAVORITE WORKOUTS

After each chapter, Coach Ben offers a pro tip describing his favorite workout for that event distance. Most of these workouts feature mixed intensities and are different from the run types detailed in this overview. Entire training plans designed by Coach Ben are available in interactive format at nazelite.com.

Online versions of the plans in this book—plus a beginner-friendly level 0 plan for each race distance—are available at 8020endurance .com. Adaptive versions that are customized to the individual and continuously adjust based on your availability and progress are available through the PACE smartphone app. By no means do these training plans encapsulate all that it means to run like a pro. But having read this far, you know that already. What it truly means to run like a pro is to experience the most fulfilling journey possible as a runner by matching your passion for the sport with the best and most efficient methods of unlocking the potential of any runner, regardless of experience or ability. Enjoy every minute of it!

10

5K TRAINING PLANS

*T*HE 5K IS THE only popular road running event that is performed at high intensity (i.e., above critical velocity) by most runners. Success at this distance therefore requires that you do plenty of work at high intensity in training. But it's still a distance event, not a sprint—more than 90 percent of the energy required to cover 3.1 miles as quickly as possible comes from aerobic rather than anaerobic metabolism—so you mustn't neglect aerobic development when you're focused on the 5K.

The three pro-style training plans presented in this chapter offer the right balance of low, moderate, and high intensities for optimal 5K performance. The level 1 plan features four runs per week, plus two sessions that may be done either as easy runs or as nonimpact cardio cross-training sessions, and one rest day. You should be able to run comfortably for at least forty minutes at a time before you begin this plan. The level 2 plan features seven runs per week (six in recovery weeks), and you should be running daily for up to seventy minutes before you begin. Finally, the level 3 plan features nine runs per week (eight in recovery weeks), and you should have a solid fitness base that includes daily running and some work at higher intensities before you start it.

All three plans contain three-week step cycles, where the training load is reduced for recovery in the third week. Refer back to the Training Plans Overview for details on how to do the various workout types. Coach Ben's favorite 5K workout follows this chapter. Interactive, online versions of these training plans—plus a beginner-friendly level 0 plan—are available at 8020endurance.com. Adaptive versions are available through the PACE smartphone app.

· LEVEL 1 ·

	MONDAY	TUESDAY	WEDNESDAY	THURSDAY	FRIDAY	SATURDAY	SUNDAY
1	Rest	Fartlek Run 10:00 easy Drills and Strides 6 x (0:20 @ VHI/1:40 easy) 5:00 easy	Easy Run or Cross-Training 30:00 easy	Easy Run 30:00 easy	Fast-Finish Run 25:00 easy 5:00 @ CV	Easy Run or Cross-Training 30:00 easy	Long Run 40:00 easy
2	Rest	Fartlek Run 10:00 easy Drills and Strides 6 x (1:00 @ MAS/2:00 easy) 10:00 easy	Easy Run or Cross-Training 30:00 easy	Easy Run 30:00 easy	Fast-Finish Run 25:00 easy 10:00 @ LTP	Easy Run or Cross-Training 30:00 easy	Long Run 50:00 easy
3	Rest	Hill-Repetitions Run 10:00 easy Drills and Strides 8 x (0:30 uphill @ VHI/1:130 easy) 10:00 easy	Easy Run or Cross-Training 30:00 easy	Easy Run 30:00 easy	Progression Run 20:00 easy 8:00 @ SSP 4:00 @ LTP 2:00 @ CV 5:00 easy	Easy Run or Cross-Training 30:00 easy	Long Run 40:00 easy
4	Rest	Descending-Intervals Run 10:00 easy Drills and Strides 3:00 @ MAS/2:00 easy 2:00 @ MAS/1:20 easy 1:00 @ MAS/0:40 easy 0:45 @ MAS/0:30 easy 0:30 @ MAS 10:00 easy	Easy Run or Cross-Training 35:00 easy	Easy Run 30:00 easy	Critical-Velocity Intervals Run 10:00 easy Drills and Strides 4 x (4:00 @ CV/2:00 easy) 10:00 easy	Easy Run or Cross-Training 35:00 easy	Long Run 1:00:00 easy

(Table continues) 211

	MONDAY	TUESDAY	WEDNESDAY	THURSDAY	FRIDAY	SATURDAY	SUNDAY
5	Rest	Lactate-Intervals Run 10:00 easy Drills and Strides 8 x (0:30 @ MAS/0:15 easy) 3:00 easy 8 x (0:30 @ MAS/0:15 easy) 8 x (0:30 @ MAS/0:15 easy) 10:00 easy	Easy Run or Cross-Training 35:00 easy	Easy Run 30:00 easy	Steady-State Run 10:00 easy 30:00 @ SSP 10:00 easy	Easy Run or Cross-Training 35:00 easy	Long Run 1:10:00 easy
6	Rest	Speed-Intervals Run 10:00 easy Drills and Strides 6 x 1:00 @ VHI/2:00 easy 10:00 easy	Easy Run or Cross-Training 35:00 easy	Easy Run 30:00 easy	Progression Run 20:00 easy 12:00 @ SSP 6:00 @ LTP 3:00 @ CV 5:00 easy	Easy Run or Cross-Training 35:00 easy	Long Run 50:00 easy
7	Rest	Variable-Speed Intervals Run 10:00 easy Drills and Strides 3 x (4 x 0:30 @ MAS/0:45 @ LTP) 2:30 easy 10:00 easy	Easy Run or Cross-Training 40:00 easy	Easy Run 30:00 easy	Tempo Run 10:00 easy Drills and Strides 14:00 @ LTP 5:00 easy 14:00 @ LTP 10:00 easy	Easy Run or Cross-Training 40:00 easy	Long Run 1:20:00 easy
8	Rest	Coach Ben's Favorite 5K Workout 1 mile easy Drills and Strides 7 x 3:00 @ CV +0:08–0:10 per mile/1:00 rest (3:00 after final rep) 1-mile time trial 1 mile easy	Easy Run or Cross-Training 40:00 easy	Easy Run 30:00 easy	Critical-Velocity Intervals Run 10:00 easy Drills and Strides 5 x (4:00 @ CV/2:00 easy) 10:00 easy	Easy Run or Cross-Training 40:00 easy	Long Run 1:00:00 easy

	MONDAY	TUESDAY	WEDNESDAY	THURSDAY	FRIDAY	SATURDAY	SUNDAY
9	Rest	Fartlek Run 10:00 easy Drills and Strides 6 x (1:00 @ MAS/2:00 easy) 10:00 easy	Easy Run or Cross-Training 35:00 easy	Fast Finish Run 25:00 easy 5:00 @ CV	Easy Run plus Strides 20:00 easy Drills and Strides	5K Race	Rest

213

• LEVEL 2 •

	MONDAY	TUESDAY	WEDNESDAY	THURSDAY	FRIDAY	SATURDAY	SUNDAY
1	Easy Run 30:00 easy	Fartlek Run 15:00 easy Drills and Strides 8 x (0:20 @ VHI/1:40 easy) 15:00 easy	Easy Run 40:00 easy	Easy Run plus Strides 1:00:00 easy Drills and Strides	Fast-Finish Run 40:00 easy 5:00 @ CV	Easy Run 40:00 easy	Long Run 1:10:00 easy
2	Easy Run 30:00 easy	Fartlek Run 15:00 easy Drills and Strides 8 x (1:00 @ MAS/2:00 easy) 15:00 easy	Easy Run 40:00 easy	Easy Run plus Strides 1:00:00 easy Drills and Strides	Fast-Finish Run 40:00 easy 10:00 @ LTP	Easy Run 40:00 easy	Steady-State Run 15:00 easy 30:00 @ SSP 15:00 easy
3	Rest	Hill-Repetitions Run 15:00 easy Drills and Strides 8 x (0:45 uphill @ VHI/1:45 easy) 15:00 easy	Easy Run 40:00 easy	Easy Run plus Strides 1:00:00 easy Drills and Strides	Progression Run 30:00 easy 8:00 @ SSP 4:00 @ LTP 2:00 @ CV 5:00 easy	Easy Run 40:00 easy	Long Run 1:20:00 easy
4	Easy Run 30:00 easy	Descending-Intervals Run 15:00 easy Drills and Strides 3:00 @ MAS/2:00 easy 2:00 @ MAS/1:20 easy 1:00 @ MAS/0:40 easy 0:45 @ MAS/0:30 easy 0:30 @ MAS/0:20 easy 0:45 @ MAS/0:30 easy 0:30 @ MAS 15:00 easy	Easy Run 45:00 easy	Easy Run plus Strides 1:00:00 easy Drills and Strides	Critical-Velocity Intervals Run 15:00 easy Drills and Strides 5 x (4:00 @ CV/2:00 easy) 15:00 easy	Easy Run 45:00 easy	Tempo Run 15:00 easy 8:00 @ LTP 5:00 easy 8:00 @ LTP 5:00 easy 8:00 @ LTP 15:00 easy

	MONDAY	TUESDAY	WEDNESDAY	THURSDAY	FRIDAY	SATURDAY	SUNDAY
5	Easy Run 30:00 easy	Lactate-Intervals Run 15:00 easy Drills and Strides 10 x (0:30 @ MAS/0:15 easy) 3:00 easy 10 x (0:30 @ MAS/0:15 easy) 10 x (0:30 @ MAS/0:15 easy) 15:00 easy	Easy Run 45:00 easy	Easy Run plus Strides 1:00:00 easy Drills and Strides	Over/Under Intervals Run 15:00 easy Drills and Strides 3 x (3:00 @ LTP plus 0:05 per mile/4:00 @ LTP-0:05 per mile/2:00 easy) 15:00 easy	Easy Run 45:00 easy	Steady-State Run 15:00 easy 40:00 @ SSP 15:00 easy
6	Rest	Leg-Speed Run 15:00 easy Drills and Strides 8 x (1:00 @ VHI/2:00 easy) 15:00 easy	Easy Run 40:00 easy	Easy Run plus Strides 1:00:00 easy Drills and Strides	Progression Run 30:00 easy 12:00 @ SSP 6:00 @ LTP 3:00 @ CV 5:00 easy	Easy Run 40:00 easy	Long Run 1:30:00 easy
7	Easy Run 30:00 easy	Variable-Speed Intervals Run 15:00 easy Drills and Strides 4 x (4 x 0:30 @ MAS/0:45 @ LTP) 2:30 easy 15:00 easy	Easy Run 50:00 easy	Easy Run plus Strides 1:00:00 easy Drills and Strides	10K Pace Intervals Run 15:00 easy Drills and Strides 10 x 1 kilometer @ 10KP/1:00 rest 15:00 easy	Easy Run 50:00 easy	Tempo Run 15:00 easy 10:00 @ LTP 5:00 easy 10:00 @ LTP 5:00 easy 10:00 @ LTP 15:00 easy

(Table continues)

	MONDAY	TUESDAY	WEDNESDAY	THURSDAY	FRIDAY	SATURDAY	SUNDAY
8	Easy Run 30:00 easy	Coach Ben's Favorite 5K Workout 15:00 easy Drills and Strides 7 x 3:00 @ CV plus 0:08–0:10 per mile/1:00 rest (3:00 after final rep) 1-mile time trial 15:00 easy	Easy Run 50:00 easy	Easy Run plus Strides 1:00:00 easy Drills and Strides	Progression-Intervals Run 15:00 easy Drills and Strides 5 x (0:30 @ SSP/0:20 @ MAS/0:10 @ VHI) 5:00 easy 5 x (0:30 @ SSP/0:20 @ MAS/0:10 @ VHI) 5:00 easy 5 x (0:30 @ SSP/0:20 @ MAS/0:10 @ VHI) 15:00 easy	Easy Run 50:00 easy	Long Run with Fast Finish 1:00:00 easy 10:00 @ LTP
9	Rest	Fartlek Run 15:00 easy Drills and Strides 8 x (1:00 @ MAS/2:00 easy) 15:00 easy	Easy Run 45:00 easy	Fast Finish Run 25:00 easy 5:00 @ CV	Easy Run plus Strides 20:00 easy Drills and Strides	5K Race	Rest

· LEVEL 3 ·

	MONDAY	TUESDAY	WEDNESDAY	THURSDAY	FRIDAY	SATURDAY	SUNDAY
1	Easy Run 40:00 easy	Fartlek Run 20:00 easy Drills and Strides 10 x (0:20 @ VHI/1:40 easy) 20:00 easy Easy Run 20:00 easy	Easy Run 45:00 easy	Easy Run plus Drills, Strides, and Plyos 1:00:00 easy Drills, Strides, and Plyos	Fast-Finish Run 55:00 easy 5:00 @ CV Easy Run 20:00 easy	Easy Run 45:00 easy	Long Run 1:20:00 easy
2	Easy Run 40:00 easy	Fartlek Run 20:00 easy Drills and Strides 10 x (1:00 @ MAS/2:00 easy) 20:00 easy Easy Run 20:00 easy	Easy Run 50:00 easy	Easy Run plus Drills, Strides, and Plyos 1:00:00 easy Drills, Strides, and Plyos	Fast-Finish Run 50:00 easy 10:00 @ LTP Easy Run 20:00 easy	Easy Run 50:00 easy	Steady-State Run 20:00 easy 30:00 @ SSP 20:00 easy
3	Rest	Hill-Repetitions Run 20:00 easy Drills and Strides 10 x (0:30 uphill @ VHI/1:30 easy) 20:00 easy Easy Run 20:00 easy	Easy Run 45:00 easy	Easy Run plus Drills, Strides, and Plyos 1:00:00 easy Drills, Strides, and Plyos	Progression Run 30:00 easy 12:00 @ SSP 6:00 @ LTP 3:00 @ CV 5:00 easy Easy Run 20:00 easy	Easy Run 45:00 easy	Long Run 1:40:00 easy

(Table continues)

	MONDAY	TUESDAY	WEDNESDAY	THURSDAY	FRIDAY	SATURDAY	SUNDAY
4	Easy Run 40:00 easy	Descending-Intervals Run 20:00 easy Drills and Strides 3:00 @ MAS/2:00 easy 2:00 @ MAS/1:20 easy 1:00 @ MAS/0:40 easy 0:45 @ MAS/0:30 easy 0:30 @ MAS/0:20 easy 1:00 @ MAS/0:40 easy 0:45 @ MAS/0:30 easy 0:30 @ MAS 20:00 easy Easy Run 25:00 easy	Easy Run 55:00 easy	Easy Run plus Drills, Strides, and Plyos 1:00:00 easy Drills, Strides, and Plyos	Critical-Velocity Intervals Run 20:00 easy Drills and Strides 6 x (4:00 @ CV/2:00 easy) 20:00 easy Easy Run 25:00 easy	Easy Run 55:00 easy	Tempo Run 20:00 easy 10:00 @ LTP 5:00 easy 10:00 @ LTP 5:00 easy 10:00 @ LTP 20:00 easy
5	Easy Run 40:00 easy	Lactate-Intervals Run 20:00 easy Drills and Strides 12 x (0:30 @ MAS/0:15 easy) 3:00 easy 12 x (0:30 @ MAS/0:15 easy) 3:00 easy 12 x (0:30 @ MAS/0:15 easy) 20:00 easy Easy Run 25:00 easy	Easy Run 1:00:00 easy	Easy Run plus Drills, Strides, and Plyos 1:00:00 easy Drills, Strides, and Plyos	Over/Under Intervals Run 20:00 easy Drills and Strides 4 x (3:00 @ LTP plus 0:05 per mile/3:00 @ LTP-0:05 per mile/3:00 easy) 20:00 easy Easy Run 25:00 easy	Easy Run 1:00:00 easy	Steady-State Run 20:00 easy 40:00 @ SSP 20:00 easy

	MONDAY	TUESDAY	WEDNESDAY	THURSDAY	FRIDAY	SATURDAY	SUNDAY
6	Rest	Leg-Speed Run 20:00 easy Drills and Strides 10 x (1:00 @ VHI/2:00 easy) 20:00 easy Easy Run 25:00 easy	Easy Run 50:00 easy	Easy Run plus Drills, Strides, and Plyos 1:00:00 easy Drills, Strides, and Plyos	Progression Run 30:00 easy 16:00 @ SSP 8:00 @ LTP 4:00 @ CV 5:00 easy Easy Run 25:00 easy	Easy Run 50:00 easy	Long Run 2:00:00 easy
7	Easy Run 40:00 easy	Variable-Speed Intervals Run 20:00 easy Drills and Strides 5 x (4 x 0:30 @ MAS/0:45 @ LTP) 2:30 easy 20:00 easy Easy Run 30:00 easy	Easy Run 1:00:00 easy	Easy Run plus Drills, Strides, and Plyos 1:00:00 easy Drills, Strides, and Plyos	10K Pace Intervals Run 20:00 easy Drills and Strides 10 x 1 kilometer @ 10KP/1:00 rest 20:00 easy Easy Run 30:00 easy	Easy Run 1:00:00 easy	Tempo Run 20:00 easy 12:00 @ LTP 5:00 easy 12:00 @ LTP 5:00 easy 12:00 @ LTP 20:00 easy

(Table continues)

	MONDAY	TUESDAY	WEDNESDAY	THURSDAY	FRIDAY	SATURDAY	SUNDAY
8	Easy Run 40:00 easy	Coach Ben's Favorite 5K Workout 20:00 easy Drills and Strides 7 x 3:00 @ CV plus 0:08–0:10 per mile/1:00 rest (3:00 after final rep) 1-mile time trial 20:00 easy Easy Run 30:00 easy	Easy Run 1:00:00 easy	Easy Run plus Drills, Strides, and Plyos 1:00:00 easy Drills, Strides, and Plyos	Progression-Intervals Run 20:00 easy Drills and Strides 5 x (0:30 @ SSP/0:20 @ MAS/0:10 @ VHI) 5:00 easy 5 x (0:30 @ SSP/0:20 @ MAS/0:10 @ VHI) 5:00 easy 5 x (0:30 @ SSP/0:20 @ MAS/0:10 @ VHI) 5:00 easy 5 x (0:30 @ SSP/0:20 @ MAS/0:10 @ VHI) 20:00 easy Easy Run 30:00 easy	Easy Run 1:00:00 easy	Long Run with Fast Finish 1:10:00 easy 10:00 @ LTP
9	Rest	Fartlek Run 20:00 easy Drills and Strides 10 x (1:00 @ MAS/2:00 easy) 20:00 easy	Easy Run 1:00:00 easy	Fast-Finish Run 35:00 easy 5:00 @ CV	Easy Run plus Strides 20:00 easy Drills and Strides	5K Race	Rest

My Favorite 5K Workout

7 x 3:00 at forty-five-minute pace (critical velocity plus eight to ten seconds per mile) with 1:00 rest (3:00 rest after the last rep) plus 1 x 1-mile time trial

B elieve it or not, my favorite 5K workout does not involve any targeted work at 5K race pace. Blasphemy, right? But here's the deal: time and time again, from my own running days, to my days of working with high school cross-country runners, to my present work coaching professionals who make a living based on their results, I have found that athletes typically run their fastest 5K races without doing a whole lot of traditional, ball-buster 5K-specific workouts, like 3 x 1 mile or 5 x 1K or 6 x 800 at goal 5K race pace. These workouts are fine every once in a while, but in my experience they often leave athletes feeling totally wrecked, or "flat."

Sure, you can make them somewhat less ball-busting by including long rest periods between reps, but last I checked, you don't get to take a break in a 5K. You don't get to stop halfway through and wait until your heart rate returns to its resting state before you get going again. No, in a 5K, you are running at the high end of what I call comfortably uncomfortable nearly the entire way. So workouts with giant rest intervals do not make a ton of sense to me during training for this event, or any distance above the mile, really.

I prefer workouts at actual 5K pace to be low in distance per repeat but high in the total number of repetitions. So, things like 20–30 x 200 at 5K pace or 16–20 x 300 at 5K pace with a 100–200-meter jog between reps. But even these workouts should be done sparingly in 5K training. The bulk of the workouts in a 5K training segment should be no different than what you do to get fit for any distance—things like fast-finish long runs, 8–15 x 1K at threshold pace, and 16–20 x 400 meters at critical velocity. That being said, I do like to modify these workouts in the lead-up to a 5K by tacking on a half mile to a mile's worth of some short reps at one-mile race pace after the rest of the session has been completed. You might want to do 10 x 100, or 8 x 200, or 4 x 300. These final portions of the workout are a great way to work on smooth, fast running on tired legs. And they serve as a prerequisite for the workout I am about to describe.

Let's say that, over the course of twelve to twenty weeks, you've done all the things I've described, and you've kept your mileage in your sweet spot, and you've got a 5K coming up in about ten days. My absolute favorite workout in this situation for the pros I coach consists of 7 x 1K at a pace that's roughly their 15K race pace with a minute's rest between repetitions. The pace is just fast enough to provide a good stimulus and put a little bit of fatigue into their legs, while the recovery is short enough to keep their heart rate high throughout. Then, we triple the rest after repeat number seven and let them loose for an all-out mile. The first time I tried this workout was in 2017 with two male athletes who were getting ready for a 5K on the track. They ran their 1K repeats in 2:55 with relative ease, and then ran the all-out mile in 4:16. Nine days later, they ran 13:29 (4:20 per mile pace) and 13:36 (4:22 per mile pace) for 5000 meters.

Both of the athletes really enjoyed the session (and I'm a big believer that the more enjoyable training is, the more effective it is), and of course it was hard to argue with the results. The reason I like this workout is that it has you running the all-out mile in a state of fatigue. Sure, you aren't quite as fatigued as you'll be in the last mile of a 5K, but you're not as fresh as you'll be in the first mile, either. I believe the first three-quarters of the time trial closely simulate how you'll feel in the middle mile of the 5K, and the last quarter probably feels fairly similar to the last quarter-mile of the 5K itself. So, even though you're not consciously targeting your 5K pace, the workout should leave you feeling physically and mentally prepared for your upcoming 5K race.

I'll let you decide for yourself how enjoyable it is.

222

11

10K TRAINING PLANS

*I*F I WANTED TO know how fit a given runner was, and I had to base my assessment on a single piece of information, I would want to know that person's 10K time. That's because the 10K demands a more balanced blend of the various components of running fitness, from speed to stamina, than any other race distance. If you can run a solid 10K, you can also run a strong 1500 meters or a successful marathon. For proof, look at pros like Sifan Hassan, who won both the 1500 meters and the 10,000 meters for the Netherlands at the 2019 World Outdoor Championships, and Galen Rupp, who doubled at 10,000 meters and the marathon at the 2016 Olympics, finishing fifth in the former event and taking the bronze medal in the latter.

No matter what your favorite event is, you'll get better at it if you get better at the 10K, and the three training plans presented in this chapter will help you do just that. The level 1 plan features four runs per week, plus two sessions that may be done either as easy runs or as nonimpact cardio cross-training sessions, and a rest day. You should be able to run comfortably for at least an hour before you begin this plan. The level 2 plan features seven runs per week (six in recovery weeks), and you should be running daily for up to eighty minutes before you begin. Finally, the level 3 plan features nine runs per week (eight in recovery weeks), and you should have a solid fitness base that includes daily running and some work at higher intensities before you start it.

All three plans contain three-week step cycles, where the training load is reduced for recovery in the third week. Refer back to the Training Plans Overview for details on how to do the various workout types. Coach Ben's favorite 10K workout is described in a pro tip that follows this chapter. Interactive, online versions of these training plans—plus a beginner-friendly level 0 10K plan—are available at 8020endurance.com. Adaptive versions are available through the PACE smartphone app.

• LEVEL 1 •

	MONDAY	TUESDAY	WEDNESDAY	THURSDAY	FRIDAY	SATURDAY	SUNDAY
1	Rest	Fast-Finish Run 35:00 easy 5:00 @ CV	Easy Run or Cross-Training 30:00 easy	Easy Run 30:00 easy	Fartlek Run 10:00 easy Drills and Strides 6 x 0:20 @ MAS/1:40 easy 10:00 easy	Easy Run or Cross-Training 30:00 easy	Long Run 1:05:00 easy
2	Rest	Fast-Finish Run 30:00 easy 10:00 @ LTP	Easy Run or Cross-Training 35:00 easy	Easy Run 35:00 easy	Fartlek Run 10:00 easy Drills and Strides 6 x 1:00 @ MAS/2:00 easy 10:00 easy	Easy Run or Cross-Training 35:00 easy	Long Run 1:10:00 easy
3	Rest	Fartlek Run 10:00 easy Drills and Strides 1:00 @ 5KP 1:00 easy 2:00 @ 10KP 1:00 easy 3:00 @ HMP 1:00 easy 2:00 @ 10KP 1:00 easy 1:00 @ 5KP 10:00 easy	Easy Run or Cross-Training 30:00 easy	Easy Run 30:00 easy	Hill-Repetitions Run 10:00 easy Drills and Strides 6 x 0:30 uphill @ VHI/1:30 easy 10:00 easy	Easy Run or Cross-Training 30:00 easy	Long Run 1:05:00 easy

	MONDAY	TUESDAY	WEDNESDAY	THURSDAY	FRIDAY	SATURDAY	SUNDAY
4	Rest	Critical-Velocity Intervals Run 10:00 easy 4 x 4:00 @ CV/2:00 easy 10:00 easy	Easy Run or Cross-Training 35:00 easy	Easy Run 40:00 easy	Variable-Speed Intervals Run 10:00 easy Drills and Strides 3 x (4 x 0:30 @ MAS/0:45 @ LTP) 2:30 easy 10:00 easy	Easy Run or Cross-Training 35:00 easy	Long Run 1:15:00 easy
5	Rest	Steady-State Run 10:00 easy 30:00 @ SSP 10:00 easy	Easy Run or Cross-Training 40:00 easy	Easy Run 45:00 easy	Accelerations Run 10:00 easy Drills and Strides 11:00 acceleration from jog to sprint 10:00 walk to jog 3:00 acceleration from jog to sprint 10:00 walk to jog	Easy Run or Cross-Training 40:00 easy	Long Run 1:20:00 easy
6	Rest	Progression Run 20:00 easy 8:00 @ SSP 4:00 @ LTP 2:00 @ CV 5:00 easy	Easy Run or Cross-Training 35:00 easy	Easy Run 35:00 easy	Speed-Intervals Run 10:00 easy Drills and Strides 8 x 0:45 @ VHI/1:45 easy 10:00 easy	Easy Run or Cross-Training 35:00 easy	Long Run 1:10:00 easy
7	Rest	Over/Under Intervals Run 10:00 easy Drills and Strides 3 x 3:00 @ LTP plus 0:05 per mile/3:00 @ LTP-0:05 per mile/3:00 easy 10:00 easy	Easy Run or Cross-Training 40:00 easy	Easy Run 50:00 easy	Descending-Intervals Run 10:00 easy Drills and Strides 3:00 @ MAS/2:00 easy 2:00 @ MAS/1:20 easy 1:00 @ MAS/0:40 easy 0:45 @ MAS/0:30 easy 0:30 @ MAS/0:20 Easy 0:45 @ MAS/0:30 easy 0:30 @ MAS 10:00 easy	Easy Run or Cross-Training 40:00 easy	Long Run 1:25:00 easy

(Table continues)

	MONDAY	TUESDAY	WEDNESDAY	THURSDAY	FRIDAY	SATURDAY	SUNDAY
8	Rest	Tempo Run 10:00 easy 14:00 @ LTP 5:00 easy 14:00 @ LTP 10:00 easy	Easy Run or Cross-Training 45:00 easy	Easy Run 55:00 easy	Lactate-Intervals run 10:00 easy Drills and Strides 8 x (0:30 @ MAS/0:15 easy) 3:00 easy 8 x (0:30 @ MAS/0:15 easy) 3:00 easy 8 x (0:30 @ MAS/0:15 easy) 10:00 easy Speed-Intervals Run 10:00 easy Drills and Strides 8 x 1:00 @ VHI/2:00 easy 10:00 easy	Easy Run or Cross-Training 45:00 easy	Long Run 1:30:00 easy
9	Rest	Fartlek Run 10:00 easy Drills and Strides 1:00 @ 5KP 1:00 easy 2:00 @ 10KP 1:00 easy 3:00 @ HMP 1:00 easy 2:00 @ 10KP 1:00 easy 1:00 @ 5KP 1:00 easy 2:00 @ 10KP 1:00 easy 3:00 @ HMP 10:00 easy	Easy Run or Cross-Training 40:00 easy	Easy Run 40:00 easy	Progression Intervals Run 10:00 easy Drills and Strides 5 x (0:30 @ SSP/0:20 @ MAS/0:10 @ VHI) 5:00 easy 5 x (0:30 @ SSP/0:20 @ MAS/0:10 @ VHI) 5:00 easy 5 x (0:30 @ SSP/0:20 @ MAS/0:10 @ VHI) 10:00 easy	Easy Run or Cross-Training 40:00 easy	Long Run 1:15:00 easy
10	Rest	Critical-Velocity Intervals Run 10:00 easy 5 x 4:00 @ CV/2:00 easy 10:00 easy	Easy Run or Cross-Training 45:00 easy	Easy Run 1:00:00 easy	5K Pace Intervals Run 1 mile easy Drills and Strides 8 x 600 meters @ 5KP/400 meters easy 1 mile easy	Easy Run or Cross-Training 45:00 easy	Long Run 1:40:00 easy

	MONDAY	TUESDAY	WEDNESDAY	THURSDAY	FRIDAY	SATURDAY	SUNDAY
11	Rest	Coach Ben's Favorite 10K Workout 10:00 easy Drills and Strides 8 x 3:00 @ CV/1:00 rest 4 x 300 meters VHI*/1:00 rest 10:00 easy *Run each rep faster than the previous	Easy Run or Cross-Training 45:00 easy	Easy Run 1:00:00 easy	Progression Run 30:00 easy 8:00 @ LTP 4:00 @ CV 2:00 @ MAS 5:00 easy	Easy Run or Cross-Training 45:00 easy	Long Run 1:15:00 easy
12	Rest	Fast-Finish Run 40:00 easy 5:00 @ CV	Easy Run or Cross-Training 40:00 easy	Fartlek Run 10:00 easy Drills and Strides 6 x 1:00 @ MAS/2:00 easy 10:00 easy	Easy Run plus Strides 20:00 easy Drills and Strides	10K Race	Rest

227

	MONDAY	TUESDAY	WEDNESDAY	THURSDAY	FRIDAY	SATURDAY	SUNDAY
1	Easy Run 30:00 easy	Fast-Finish Run 40:00 easy 5:00 @ CV	Easy Run 45:00 easy	Easy Run plus Strides 45:00 easy Drills and Strides	Fartlek Run 15:00 easy Drills and Strides 8 x (0:20 @ VHI/1:40 easy) 15:00 easy	Easy Run 45:00 easy	Long Run 1:20:00 easy
2	Easy Run 30:00 easy	Fast-Finish Run 35:00 easy 10:00 @ LTP	Easy Run 45:00 easy	Easy Run plus Strides 45:00 easy Drills and Strides	Fartlek Run 15:00 easy Drills and Strides 8 x (1:00 @ MAS/2:00 easy) 15:00 easy	Easy Run 45:00 easy	Long Run 1:40:00 easy
3	Rest	Fartlek Run 15:00 easy Drills and Strides 1:00 @ 5KP 1:00 easy 2:00 @ 10KP 1:00 easy 3:00 @ HMP 1:00 easy 2:00 @ 10KP 1:00 easy 1:00 @ 5KP 1:00 easy 2:00 @ 10KP 1:00 easy 5:00 @ HMP 15:00 easy	Easy Run 45:00 easy	Easy Run plus Strides 45:00 easy Drills and Strides	Hill Repetitions Run 15:00 easy Drills and Strides 8 x (0:30 uphill @ VHI/1:30 easy) 15:00 easy	Easy Run 45:00 easy	Long Run 1:20:00 easy

	MONDAY	TUESDAY	WEDNESDAY	THURSDAY	FRIDAY	SATURDAY	SUNDAY
4	Easy Run 30:00 easy	Critical-Velocity Intervals Run 15:00 easy 5 x (4:00 @ CV/2:00 easy) 15:00 easy	Easy Run 50:00 easy	Easy Run plus Strides 50:00 easy Drills and Strides	Descending-Intervals Run 15:00 easy Drills and Strides 3:00 @ MAS/2:00 easy 2:00 @ MAS/1:20 easy 1:00 @ MAS/0:40 easy 0:45 @ MAS/0:30 easy 0:30 @ MAS/0:20 Easy 1:00 @ MAS/0:40 easy 0:45 @ MAS/0:30 easy 0:30 @ MAS 15:00 easy	Easy Run 50:00 easy	Steady-State Run 20:00 easy 35:00 @ SSP 20:00 easy
5	Easy Run 30:00 easy	Tempo Run 15:00 easy 14:00 @ LTP 5:00 easy 14:00 @ LTP 15:00 easy	Easy Run 50:00 easy	Easy Run plus Strides 50:00 easy Drills and Strides	Accelerations Run 15:00 easy Drills and Strides 11:00 acceleration from jog to sprint 10:00 walk to jog 6:00 acceleration from jog to sprint 15:00 walk to jog	Easy Run 50:00 easy	Half-Marathon Pace Run 2 miles easy 3 x 2 miles @ HMP/1:00 rest 2 miles easy
6	Rest	Progression Run 20:00 easy 12:00 @ SSP 6:00 @ LTP 3:00 @ CV 5:00 easy	Easy Run 50:00 easy	Easy Run plus Strides 50:00 easy Drills and Strides	Speed-Intervals Run 15:00 easy Drills and Strides 10 x 0:45 @ VHI/1:45 easy 15:00 easy	Easy Run 50:00 easy	Long Run 2:00:00 easy

(Table continues)

RUN LIKE A PRO (EVEN IF YOU'RE SLOW)

	MONDAY	TUESDAY	WEDNESDAY	THURSDAY	FRIDAY	SATURDAY	SUNDAY
7	Easy Run 30:00 easy	Over/Under Intervals Run 15:00 easy Drills and Strides 3 x (3:00 @ LTP plus 0:05 per mile/4:00 @ LTP-0:05 per mile/2:00 easy) 15:00 easy	Easy Run 55:00 easy	Easy Run plus Strides 55:00 easy Drills and Strides	Variable-Speed Intervals Run 15:00 easy Drills and Strides 4 x (4 x 0:30 @ MAS/0:45 @ LTP) 2:30 easy 15:00 easy	Easy Run 55:00 easy	Long Run with Surges 20:00 easy 10 x (1:00 @ CV/4:00 easy) 20:00 easy
8	Easy Run 30:00 easy	Critical-Velocity Intervals Run 15:00 easy 6 x (4:00 @ CV/2:00 easy) 15:00 easy	Easy Run 55:00 easy	Easy Run plus Strides 55:00 easy Drills and Strides	Lactate-Intervals run 15:00 easy Drills and Strides 10 x (0:30 @ MAS/0:15 easy) 3:00 easy 10 x (0:30 @ MAS/0:15 easy) 3:00 easy 10 x (0:30 @ MAS/0:15 easy) 15:00 easy	Easy Run 55:00 easy	Steady-State Run 20:00 easy 45:00 @ SSP 20:00 easy
9	Rest	Fartlek Run 15:00 easy Drills and Strides 1:00 @ 5KP 1:00 easy 2:00 @ 10KP 1:00 easy 3:00 @ HMP 1:00 easy 2:00 @ 10KP 1:00 easy 1:00 @ 5KP 1:00 easy 2:00 @ 10KP 1:00 easy 3:00 @ HMP 1:00 easy 2:00 @ 10KP 1:00 easy 1:00 @ 5KP 15:00 easy	Easy Run 55:00 easy	Easy Run plus Strides 55:00 easy Drills and Strides	Progression-Intervals Run 15:00 easy Drills and Strides 5 x (0:30 @ SSP/0:20 @ MAS/0:10 @ VHI) 5:00 easy 5 x (0:30 @ SSP/0:20 @ MAS/0:10 @ VHI) 5:00 easy 5 x (0:30 @ SSP/0:20 @ MAS/0:10 @ VHI) 15:00 easy	Easy Run 55:00 easy	Depletion Run 2:00:00 easy No calories before or during

	MONDAY	TUESDAY	WEDNESDAY	THURSDAY	FRIDAY	SATURDAY	SUNDAY
10	Easy Run 30:00 easy	Tempo Run 15:00 easy 16:00 @ LTP 5:00 easy 16:00 @ LTP 15:00 easy	Easy Run 1:00:00 easy	Easy Run plus Strides 1:00:00 easy Drills and Strides	5K Pace Intervals Run 2 miles easy Drills and Strides 8 x 600m @ 5KP/400 meters easy 2 miles easy	Easy Run 1:00:00 easy	Half-Marathon Pace Run 2 miles easy 2 x 3 miles @ HMP/1:00 rest 2 miles easy
11	Easy Run 30:00 easy	Coach Ben's Favorite 10K Workout 15:00 easy Drills and Strides 8 x 3:00 @ CV/1:00 rest 4 x 300 meters VHI*/1:00 rest 15:00 easy *Run each rep faster than the previous	Easy Run 1:00:00 easy	Easy Run plus Strides 1:00:00 easy Drills and Strides	Progression Run 30:00 easy 12:00 @ LTP 6:00 @ CV 3:00 @ MAS 5:00 easy	Easy Run 1:00:00 easy	Long Run 1:20:00 easy
12	Rest	Fast-Finish Run 50:00 easy 10:00 @ LTP	Easy Run 45:00 easy	Fartlek Run 15:00 easy 6 x 1:00 @ MAS/2:00 easy 15:00 easy	Easy Run plus Strides 20:00 easy Drills and Strides	10K Race	Rest

231

· LEVEL 3 ·

	MONDAY	TUESDAY	WEDNESDAY	THURSDAY	FRIDAY	SATURDAY	SUNDAY
1	Easy Run 40:00 easy	Fast-Finish Run 55:00 easy 5:00 @ CV Easy Run 20:00 easy	Easy Run 45:00 easy	Easy Run plus Drills, Strides, and Plyos 1:00:00 easy Drills, Strides, and Plyos	Fartlek Run 20:00 easy Drills and Strides 10 x (0:20 @ VHI/1:4 easy) 20:00 easy Easy Run 20:00 easy	Easy Run 45:00 easy	Long Run 1:40:00 easy
2	Easy Run 40:00 easy	Fast-Finish Run 50:00 easy 10:00 @ LTP Easy Run 25:00 easy	Easy Run 50:00 easy	Easy Run plus Drills, Strides, and Plyos 1:00:00 easy Drills, Strides, and Plyos	Fartlek Run 20:00 easy Drills and Strides 10 x (1:00 @ MAS/2:00 easy) 20:00 easy Easy Run 25:00 easy	Easy Run 50:00 easy	Long Run 2:00:00 easy
3	Rest	Progression Run 30:00 easy 12:00 @ SSP 6:00 @ LTP 3:00 @ CV 5:00 easy Easy Run 20:00 easy	Easy Run 45:00 easy	Easy Run plus Drills, Strides, and Plyos 1:00:00 easy Drills, Strides, and Plyos	Hill-Repetitions Run 20:00 easy Drills and Strides 10 x (0:30 uphill @ VHI/1:30 easy) 20:00 easy Easy Run 20:00 easy	Easy Run 45:00 easy	Long Run 1:40:00 easy

	MONDAY	TUESDAY	WEDNESDAY	THURSDAY	FRIDAY	SATURDAY	SUNDAY
4	Easy Run 40:00 easy	Critical-Velocity Intervals Run 20:00 easy 6 x (4:00 @ CV/2:00 easy) 20:00 easy	Easy Run 55:00 easy	Easy Run plus Drills, Strides, and Plyos 1:00:00 easy Drills, Strides, and Plyos	Descending-Intervals Run 20:00 easy Drills and Strides 3:00 @ MAS/2:00 easy 2:00 @ MAS/1:20 easy 1:00 @ MAS/0:40 easy 0:45 @ MAS/0:30 easy 0:30 @ MAS/0:20 Easy 2:00 @ MAS/1:20 easy 1:00 @ MAS/0:40 easy 0:45 @ MAS/0:30 easy 0:30 @ MAS/0:20 Easy 0:45 @ MAS/0:30 easy 0:30 @ MAS 20:00 easy	Easy Run 55:00 easy	Fast-Finish Run 1:10:00 easy 10:00 @ LTP
		Easy Run 25:00 easy			Easy Run 25:00 easy		
5	Easy Run 40:00 easy	Tempo Run 20:00 easy 14:00 @ LTP 5:00 easy 14:00 @ LTP 20:00 easy	Easy Run 1:00:00 easy	Easy Run plus Drills, Strides, and Plyos 1:00:00 easy Drills, Strides, and Plyos	Analog-Accelerations Run 20:00 easy 11:00 acceleration from jog to sprint 10:00 walk to jog 6:00 acceleration from jog to sprint 10:00 walk to jog 3:00 acceleration from jog to sprint 20:00 walk to jog	Easy Run 1:00:00 easy	Steady-State Run 20:00 easy 40:00 @ SSP 20:00 easy
		Easy Run 30:00 easy			Easy Run 30:00 easy		

RUN LIKE A PRO (EVEN IF YOU'RE SLOW)

	MONDAY	TUESDAY	WEDNESDAY	THURSDAY	FRIDAY	SATURDAY	SUNDAY
6	Rest	Fartlek Run 20:00 easy Drills and Strides 1:00 @ 5KP 1:00 easy 2:00 @ 10KP 1:00 easy 3:00 @ HMP 1:00 easy 2:00 @ 10KP 1:00 easy 1:00 @ 5KP 1:00 easy 2:00 @ 10KP 1:00 easy 3:00 @ HMP 1:00 easy 2:00 @ 10KP 1:00 easy 1:00 @ 5KP 20:00 easy	Easy Run 50:00 easy	Easy Run plus Drills, Strides, and Plyos 1:00:00 easy Drills, Strides, and Plyos	Speed-Intervals Run 20:00 easy Drills and Strides 12 x 0:45 @ VHI/1:45 easy 20:00 easy	Easy Run 50:00 easy	Long Run 2:00:00 easy
		Easy Run 25:00 easy			Easy Run 25:00 easy		
7	Easy Run 40:00 easy	Over/Under Intervals Run 20:00 easy Drills and Strides 4 x (3:00 @ LTP plus 0:05 per mile/3:00 @ LTP-0:05 per mile/3:00 easy) 20:00 easy	Easy Run 1:00:00 easy	Easy Run plus Drills, Strides, and Plyos 1:00:00 easy Drills, Strides, and Plyos	Variable-Speed Intervals Run 20:00 easy Drills and Strides 5 x (4 x 0:30 @ MAS/0:45 @ LTP) 2:30 easy 20:00 easy	Easy Run 1:00:00 easy	Half-Marathon Pace Run 3 miles easy 3 x 2 miles @ HMP/1:00 rest 3 miles easy
		Easy Run 30:00 easy			Easy Run 30:00 easy		

	MONDAY	TUESDAY	WEDNESDAY	THURSDAY	FRIDAY	SATURDAY	SUNDAY
8	Easy Run 40:00 easy	Critical-Velocity Intervals Run 20:00 easy 7 x (4:00 @ CV/2:00 easy) 20:00 easy Easy Run 30:00 easy	Easy Run 1:00:00 easy	Easy Run plus Drills, Strides, and Plyos 1:00:00 easy Drills, Strides, and Plyos	Lactate-Intervals run 20:00 easy Drills and Strides 12 x (0:30 @ MAS/0:15 easy) 3:00 easy 12 x (0:30 @ MAS/0:15 easy) 3:00 easy 12 x (0:30 @ MAS/0:15 easy) 20:00 easy Easy Run 30:00 easy	Easy Run 1:00:00 easy	Fast Finish Run 1:20:00 easy 10:00 @ LTP
9	Rest	Progression Run 30:00 easy 16:00 @ SSP 8:00 @ LTP 4:00 @ CV 5:00 easy Easy Run 30:00 easy	Easy Run 55:00 easy	Easy Run plus Drills, Strides, and Plyos 1:00:00 easy Drills, Strides, and Plyos	Progression-Intervals Run 20:00 easy Drills and Strides 5 x (0:30 @ SSP/0:20 @ MAS/0:10 @ VHI) 5:00 easy 5 x (0:30 @ SSP/0:20 @ MAS/0:10 @ VHI) 5:00 easy 5 x (0:30 @ SSP/0:20 @ MAS/0:10 @ VHI) 5:00 easy 5 x (0:30 @ SSP/0:20 @ MAS/0:10 @ VHI) 20:00 easy Easy Run 30:00 easy	Easy Run 55:00 easy	Long Run 2:00:00 easy

(Table continues)

	MONDAY	TUESDAY	WEDNESDAY	THURSDAY	FRIDAY	SATURDAY	SUNDAY
10	Easy Run 40:00 easy	Critical-Velocity Intervals Run 20:00 easy 7 x (4:00 @ CV/2:00 easy) 20:00 easy Easy Run 30:00 easy	Easy Run 1:00:00 easy	Easy Run plus Drills, Strides, and Plyos 1:00:00 easy Drills, Strides, and Plyos	5K Pace Intervals Run 3 miles easy Drills and Strides 8 x 600 meters @ 5KP/400 meters easy 3 miles easy Easy Run 30:00 easy	Easy Run 1:00:00 easy	Steady-State Run 20:00 easy 50:00 @ SSP 20:00 easy
11	Easy Run 40:00 easy	10K Pace Intervals Run 3 miles easy 6 x 1 mile @ 10KP/ 1:00 rest 3 miles easy Easy Run 30:00 easy	Easy Run 1:00:00 easy	Easy Run plus Drills, Strides, and Plyos 1:00:00 easy Drills, Strides, and Plyos	Progression Run 30:00 easy 12:00 @ LTP 6:00 @ CV 3:00 @ MAS 5:00 easy Easy Run 30:00 easy	Easy Run 1:00:00 easy	Long Run 1:30:00 easy
12	Rest	Fast-Finish Run 50:00 easy 10:00 @ CV	Easy Run 45:00 easy	Fartlek Run 20:00 easy Drill and Strides 8 x 1:00 @ MAS/2:00 easy 20:00 easy	Easy Run + Strides 20:00 easy Drills and Strides	10K Race	Rest

Coach's Tip

My Favorite 10K Workout

8 x 3:00 at critical velocity with 1:00 rest (3:00–5:00 rest after last rep) plus 4 x 300 meters cutdown with 1:00 rest

I love the 10K. And because I do, I'm sad that it has somewhat fallen out of favor in the road-racing scene, replaced with half-marathons—a "sexier" event—and the 5K, an "easier" event. Back in the day, 10Ks were commonplace, with nearly every city hosting one as a premier event on the local running calendar. They haven't all disappeared, of course. The BOLDERBoulder, held on Memorial Day in Boulder, Colorado, and the Peachtree Road Race, which takes place on July Fourth in Atlanta, Georgia, are two of the biggest races in the entire world. I've been to both many times and can attest that each offers an experience that is well worth the suffering it dishes out via altitude (Boulder), humidity (Atlanta), and hills (both).

But I'm guessing that you don't shy away from challenges. And If I'm right about that, then the 10K is an event you should absolutely try (if you haven't already) or master (if you have tried it). Once you've made the decision to embrace this challenge, however, you need to be prepared for its specific demands. Which brings us to my favorite 10K workout, a session almost as scary as the race itself: 8 x 3 minutes at critical velocity (thirty-minute race pace) plus 4 x 300 meters.

In the preceding tip, I told you that training for the 5K, in my opinion, isn't really that different from training for all the other traditional distance races. The same point applies here. At NAZ Elite, preparing for anything from the 5K to the half-marathon involves similar training. But there are certain sessions that I like to use in the final few weeks that differ just a bit, and are a hair more specific to a certain race distance. In the case of the 10K, an event we have had a lot of success with, the workout I am about to describe does a better job than any other of preparing runners for its particular demands.

The pros usually run the workout by distance rather than time. Specifically, they do 10 x 1K instead of 8 x 3 minutes. It so happens that it takes the pros about three minutes to complete each rep (the men a little less, the women a little more), adding up to thirty or so total minutes of running at a pace they could sustain for thirty minutes straight in a race. Unless you're as fast as the pros, though, you're better off doing a time-based version of the workout. To see why, suppose your critical velocity pace is 7:15 per mile. In this case, it would take you four and a half minutes to complete each 1K rep. Obviously, it's a lot harder to go for four and a half minutes versus just three minutes at a pace you could sustain for thirty minutes, and to do so ten times is asking for trouble. To get a workout that's truly equivalent to what the pros do, therefore, you need to convert it from distance to time.

Why three minutes, though? Think about it this way: I am asking you to run for three minutes at a pace you could hold for thirty minutes. That's akin to asking you to run for one minute at a pace you could hold for ten minutes, or for six minutes at a pace you could hold for one hour. By itself, none of these things is crazy hard. But do multiple repeats at these efforts, and the difficulty level increases. And when you do multiple repeats on short rest, the difficulty—and more important, the race specificity—increases exponentially. For the 10K, you would be hard-pressed to find a more specific challenge than 8 x 3:00 at critical velocity with 1:00 rest periods. It requires great mental concentration, your heart rate will remain high throughout the entire session, and by the end you will be running on very tired legs—just like in a 10K race.

Next question: Why the 300s at the end? Under oath, I suppose I would have to tell you that there was no scientific reason behind my trying it for the first time years ago. But try it I did, and I loved what I saw from the athletes, so I've used it ever since. I suppose my logic was that, in a 10,000-meter race on the track, 300 meters from the finish line is a great place to switch gears and unleash your final kick. In my experience, the shorter the race, the longer you have to wait. So, in a 5K it's more like 200 meters to go, and in a fast 1500 it's about 125 meters. I wanted our athletes to go into a 10,000-meter championship race knowing they could rip the last 300 meters. If my goal was to destroy them, I would ask them to rip four 300s all out, but my goal is not to destroy them but to prepare them, so instead I give them the 300s in what I call "cutdown style."

I'll use Kellyn Taylor, our women's team record holder for 10,000 meters, as an example. In the summer of 2020, two and a half weeks out from a 10K track event, I gave her the following session: 10 x 1K in 3:18 with 1:00 rest after each rep; 3:00 rest; 4 x 300 in fifty-two, fifty-one, fifty, and forty-nine seconds with 1:00 rest. (Note that we did this workout at 7,300 feet of elevation, so those 3:18s were the equivalent of 3:07s at sea level. There is no need to convert repeats shorter than 600 meters, though, so the 300s were the same paces they would have been no matter where we did them.)

Here's how I came up with Kellyn's times for each 300: I started with her mile time, about 4:30. That's fifty seconds per 300. So I made that the goal for number three. I made the first one two ticks slower, fifty-two, so we could go from fifty-two to forty-nine for the set. She nailed it. That workout was run on Friday, August 14. On Tuesday, September 1, Kellyn ran 31:07.60 for 10,000 meters (3:06.7 per kilometer).

I can't guarantee that this workout will produce such exact results for you, but I can promise that, done in the proper context, it'll be a huge challenge and a great way to prepare for your own 10K race, wherever it may be.

12

HALF-MARATHON TRAINING PLANS

*T*HE HALF-MARATHON IS PROBABLY my favorite race distance. I like that it's long enough to make me feel justified in eating whatever I want after finishing one, yet short enough that I can do them relatively frequently as compared to a marathon. I also like the training. Elite half-marathon specialists tend to prioritize workouts that are longer and a bit less intense than track specialists do, as well as long runs that are shorter and a little more intense than marathon specialists do, and as you would expect, I follow their cue when I train for 13.1-milers.

The three training plans presented in this chapter have the same emphases. The level 1 plan features four runs per week, plus two sessions that may be done either as easy runs or as nonimpact cardio cross-training sessions, and a rest day. You should be able to run comfortably for at least an hour before you begin this plan. The level 2 plan features seven runs per week (six in recovery weeks), and you should be running daily for up to eighty minutes before you begin. Finally, the level 3 plan features nine runs per week (eight in recovery weeks), and you should have a solid fitness base that includes daily running and some work at higher intensities before you start it.

All three plans contain three-week step cycles, where the training load is reduced for recovery in the third week. Refer back to the Training Plans Overview for details on how to do the various workout types. Coach Ben's favorite half-marathon workout is described in a pro tip that follows this chapter. Interactive, online versions of these training plans—plus a beginner-friendly level 0 half-marathon plan—are available at 8020endurance.com. Adaptive versions are available through the PACE smartphone app.

· LEVEL 1 ·

	MONDAY	TUESDAY	WEDNESDAY	THURSDAY	FRIDAY	SATURDAY	SUNDAY
1	Rest	Fast-Finish Run 35:00 easy 5:00 @ CV	Easy Run or Cross-Training 30:00 easy	Easy Run 30:00 easy	Fartlek Run 10:00 easy Drills and Strides 6 x 0:20 @ VHI/1:20 easy 10:00 easy	Easy Run or Cross-Training 30:00 easy	Long Run 1:00:00 easy
2	Rest	Fast-Finish Run 30:00 easy 10:00 @ LTP	Easy Run or Cross-Training 35:00 easy	Easy Run 35:00 easy	Fartlek Run 10:00 easy Drills and Strides 6 x 1:00 @ MAS/2:00 easy 10:00 easy	Easy Run or Cross-Training 35:00 easy	Long Run 1:10:00 easy
3	Rest	Fartlek Run 10:00 easy Drills and Strides 1:00 @ 5KP 1:00 easy 2:00 @ 10KP 1:00 easy 3:00 @ HMP 1:00 easy 2:00 @ 10KP 1:00 easy 1:00 @ 5KP 1:00 easy 2:00 @ 10KP 1:00 easy 3:00 @ HMP 10:00 easy	Easy Run or Cross-Training 30:00 easy	Easy Run 30:00 easy	Hill Repetitions Run 10:00 easy Drills and Strides 6 x (0:30 uphill @ VHI/1:30 easy) 10:00 easy	Easy Run or Cross-Training 30:00 easy	Long Run 1:00:00 easy
4	Rest	Critical-Velocity Intervals Run 10:00 easy Drills and Strides 4 x (4:00 @ CV/2:00 easy) 10:00 easy	Easy Run or Cross-Training 35:00 easy	Easy Run 40:00 easy	Fartlek Run 10:00 easy Drills and Strides 8 x 1:00 @ MAS/2:00 easy 10:00 easy	Easy Run or Cross-Training 35:00 easy	Long Run 1:20:00 easy

(Table continues)

	MONDAY	TUESDAY	WEDNESDAY	THURSDAY	FRIDAY	SATURDAY	SUNDAY
5	Rest	Tempo Run 10:00 easy Drills and Strides 12:00 @ LTP 5:00 easy 12:00 @ LTP 10:00 easy	Easy Run or Cross-Training 40:00 easy	Easy Run 45:00 easy	Descending-Intervals Run 10:00 easy Drills and Strides 3:00 @ MAS/2:00 easy 2:00 @ MAS/1:20 easy 1:00 @ MAS/0:40 easy 0:45 @ MAS/0:30 easy 0:30 @ MAS/0:20 0:45 @ MAS/0:30 easy 0:30 @ MAS/0:20 10:00 easy	Easy Run or Cross-Training 40:00 easy	Long Run 1:30:00 easy
6	Rest	Progression Run 20:00 easy 12:00 @ HMP 8:00 @ LTP 4:00 @ CV 5:00 easy	Easy Run or Cross-Training 35:00 easy	Easy Run 35:00 easy	Speed-Intervals Run 10:00 easy Drills and Strides 8 x 0:45 @ VHI/1:45 easy 10:00 easy	Easy Run or Cross-Training 35:00 easy	Long Run 1:10:00 easy
7	Rest	Steady-State Run 10:00 easy Drills and Strides 30:00 @ SSP 10:00 easy	Easy Run or Cross-Training 40:00 easy	Easy Run 50:00 easy	Accelerations Run 10:00 easy Drills and Strides 11:00 acceleration from jog to sprint 10:00 walk to jog 3:00 acceleration from jog to sprint 10:00 walk to jog	Easy Run or Cross-Training 40:00 easy	Half-Marathon Pace Run 1 mile easy Drills and Strides 3 x 2 miles @ HMP/1:00 rest 1 mile easy

242

	MONDAY	TUESDAY	WEDNESDAY	THURSDAY	FRIDAY	SATURDAY	SUNDAY
8	Rest	Over/Under Intervals Run 10:00 easy Drills and Strides 3 x (3:00 @ LTP plus 0:05 per mile/3:00 @ LTP-0:05 per mile/3:00 easy) 10:00 easy	Easy Run or Cross-Training 45:00 easy	Easy Run 55:00 easy	Variable-Speed Intervals Run 10:00 easy Drills and Strides 3 x (4 x 0:30 @ MAS/0:45 @ LTP) 2:30 easy 10:00 easy	Easy Run or Cross-Training 45:00 easy	Long Run 1:50:00 easy
9	Rest	Fartlek Run 10:00 easy Drills and Strides 1:00 @ 5KP 1:00 easy 2:00 @ 10KP 1:00 easy 3:00 @ HMP 1:00 easy 2:00 @ 10KP 1:00 easy 1:00 @ 5KP 1:00 easy 2:00 @ 10KP 1:00 easy 3:00 @ HMP 1:00 easy 2:00 @ 10KP 1:00 easy 1:00 @5KP 10:00 easy	Easy Run or Cross-Training 40:00 easy	Easy Run 40:00 easy	Hill-Repetitions Run 10:00 easy Drills and Strides 8 x (1:00 uphill @ VHI/2:00 easy) 10:00 easy	Easy Run or Cross-Training 40:00 easy	Long Run 1:20:00 easy
10	Rest	Critical-Velocity Intervals Run 10:00 easy Drills and Strides 4 x (4:00 @ CV/2:00 easy) 10:00 easy	Easy Run or Cross-Training 45:00 easy	Easy Run 1:00:00 easy	Lactate-Intervals Run 10:00 easy Drills and Strides 8 x (0:30 @ MAS/0:15 easy) 3:00 easy 8 x (0:30 @ MAS/0:15 easy) 8 x (0:30 @ MAS/0:15 easy) 10:00 easy	Easy Run or Cross-Training 45:00 easy	Long Run 2:00:00 easy

(Table continues)

	MONDAY	TUESDAY	WEDNESDAY	THURSDAY	FRIDAY	SATURDAY	SUNDAY
11	Rest	Tempo Run 10:00 easy Drills and Strides 14:00 @ LTP 5:00 easy 14:00 @ LTP 10:00 easy	Easy Run or Cross-Training 50:00 easy	Easy Run 1:00:00 easy	Accelerations Run 10:00 easy Drills and Strides 11:00 acceleration from jog to sprint 10:00 walk to jog 3:00 acceleration from jog to sprint 10:00 walk to jog	Easy Run or Cross-Training 50:00 easy	Long Run 2:10:00 easy
12	Rest	Progression Run 25:00 easy 12:00 @ HMP 8:00 @ LTP 4:00 @ CV 5:00 easy	Easy Run or Cross-Training 45:00 easy	Easy Run 45:00 easy	Progression- Intervals Run 10:00 easy Drills and Strides 5 x (0:30 @ SSP/0:20 @ MAS/0:10 @ VHI) 5:00 easy 5 x (0:30 @ SSP/0:20 @ MAS/0:10 @ VHI) 5:00 easy 5 x (0:30 @ SSP/0:20 @ MAS/0:10 @ VHI) 10:00 easy	Easy Run or Cross-Training 45:00 easy	Long Run 1:30:00 easy
13	Rest	Steady-State Run 10:00 easy Drills and Strides 40:00 @ SSP 10:00 easy	Easy Run or Cross-Training 50:00 easy	Easy Run 1:00:00 easy	5K Pace Intervals Run 1 mile easy Drills and Strides 8 x 600 meters @ 5KP/400 meters easy 1 mile easy	Easy Run or Cross-Training 50:00 easy	Half- Marathon Pace Run 1 mile easy Drills and Strides 8 miles @ HMP 1 mile easy

	MONDAY	TUESDAY	WEDNESDAY	THURSDAY	FRIDAY	SATURDAY	SUNDAY
14	Rest	Over/Under Intervals Run 10:00 easy Drills and Strides 4 x (3:00 @ LTP +0:05 per mile/4:00 @ LTP -0:05 per mile/2:00 easy) 10:00 easy	Easy Run or Cross-Training 50:00 easy	Easy Run 55:00 easy	Progression Run 30:00 easy 8:00 @ LTP 4:00 @ CV 2:00 @ MAS 5:00 easy	Easy Run or Cross-Training 45:00 easy	Long Run 1:20:00 easy
15	Rest	Fartlek Run 10:00 easy Drills and Strides 6 x 1:00 @ MAS/2:00 easy 10:00 easy	Easy Run or Cross-Training 40:00 easy	Easy Run 30:00 easy	Fast-Finish Run 20:00 easy 5:00 @ CV	Easy Run plus Strides 20:00 easy Drills and Strides	Half-Marathon Race

245

	MONDAY	TUESDAY	WEDNESDAY	THURSDAY	FRIDAY	SATURDAY	SUNDAY
1	Easy Run 30:00 easy	Fast-Finish Run 40:00 easy 5:00 @ CV	Easy Run 45:00 easy	Easy Run plus Strides 45:00 easy Drills and Strides	Fartlek Run 15:00 easy Drills and Strides 8 x 0:20 @ VHI/1:20 easy 15:00 easy	Easy Run 45:00 easy	Long Run 1:20:00 easy
2	Easy Run 30:00 easy	Fast Finish Run 35:00 easy 10:00 @ LTP	Easy Run 45:00 easy	Easy Run plus Strides 45:00 easy Drills and Strides	Fartlek Run 15:00 easy Drills and Strides 8 x 1:00 @ MAS/2:00 easy 15:00 easy	Easy Run 45:00 easy	Long Run 1:30:00 easy
3	Rest	Fartlek Run 15:00 easy Drills and Strides 1:00 @ 5KP 1:00 easy 2:00 @ 10KP 1:00 easy 3:00 @ HMP 1:00 easy 2:00 @ 10KP 1:00 easy 1:00 @ 5KP 1:00 easy 2:00 @ 10KP 1:00 easy 3:00 @ HMP 15:00 easy	Easy Run 45:00 easy	Easy Run plus Drills and Strides 45:00 easy Drills and Strides	Hill-Repetitions Run 15:00 easy Drills and Strides 8 x (0:30 uphill @ VHI/1:30 easy) 15:00 easy	Easy Run 45:00 easy	Long Run 1:15:00 easy
4	Easy Run 30:00 easy	Critical-Velocity Intervals Run 15:00 easy Drills and Strides 5 x (4:00 @ CV/2:00 easy) 15:00 easy	Easy Run 50:00 easy	Easy Run plus Drills and Strides 50:00 easy Drills and Strides	Fartlek Run 15:00 easy Drills and Strides 10 x 1:00 @ MAS/2:00 easy 15:00 easy	Easy Run 50:00 easy	Long Run 1:40:00 easy

	MONDAY	TUESDAY	WEDNESDAY	THURSDAY	FRIDAY	SATURDAY	SUNDAY
5	Easy Run 30:00 easy	Tempo Run 15:00 easy Drills and Strides 14:00 @ LTP 5:00 easy 14:00 @ LTP 15:00 easy	Easy Run 50:00 easy	Easy Run plus Drills and Strides 50:00 easy Drills and Strides	Descending-Intervals Run 15:00 easy Drills and Strides 3:00 @ MAS/2:00 easy 2:00 @ MAS/1:20 easy 1:00 @ MAS/0:40 easy 0:45 @ MAS/0:30 easy 0:30 @ MAS 15:00 easy	Easy Run 50:00 easy	Long Run 1:50:00 easy
6	Rest	Progression Run 20:00 easy 12:00 @ SSP 6:00 @ LTP 3:00 @ CV 5:00 easy	Easy Run 50:00 easy	Easy Run + Drills and Strides 50:00 easy Drills and Strides	Speed-Intervals Run 15:00 easy Drills and Strides 8 x (0:45 @ VHI/1:45 easy) 15:00 easy	Easy Run 50:00 easy	Long Run 1:30:00 easy
7	Easy Run 30:00 easy	Steady-State Run 15:00 easy Drills and Strides 40:00 @ SSP 15:00 easy	Easy Run 55:00 easy	Easy Run plus Drills and Strides 55:00 easy Drills and Strides	Accelerations Run 15:00 easy Drills and Strides 11:00 acceleration from jog to sprint 10:00 walk to jog 6:00 acceleration from jog to sprint 15:00 walk to jog	Easy Run 55:00 easy	Half-Marathon Pace Run 2 miles easy Drills and Strides 3 x 2 miles @ HMP/1:00 rest 2 miles easy
8	Easy Run 30:00 easy	Over/Under Intervals Run 15:00 easy Drills and Strides 3 x (3:00 @ LTP plus 0:05 per mile/4:00 @ LTP -0:05 per mile/2:00 easy) 15:00 easy	Easy Run 55:00 easy	Easy Run plus Drills and Strides 55:00 easy Drills and Strides	Variable-Speed Intervals Run 15:00 easy Drills and Strides 4 x (4 x 0:30 @ MAS/0:45 @ LTP) 2:30 easy 15:00 easy	Easy Run 55:00 easy	Long Run 2:00:00 easy

(Table continues)

	MONDAY	TUESDAY	WEDNESDAY	THURSDAY	FRIDAY	SATURDAY	SUNDAY
9	Rest	Fartlek Run 15:00 easy Drills and Strides 1:00 @ 5KP 1:00 easy 2:00 @ 10KP 1:00 easy 3:00 @ HMP 1:00 easy 2:00 @ 10KP 1:00 easy 1:00 @ 5KP 1:00 easy 2:00 @ 10KP 1:00 easy 3:00 @ HMP 15:00 easy	Easy Run 55:00 easy	Easy Run + Drills and Strides 55:00 easy Drills and Strides	Hill Repetitions Run 15:00 easy Drills and Strides 10 x (1:00 uphill @ VHI/2:00 easy) 15:00 easy	Easy Run 55:00 easy	Long Run 1:45:00 easy
10	Easy Run 30:00 easy	Critical-Velocity Intervals Run 15:00 easy 6 x (4:00 @ CV/2:00 easy) 15:00 easy	Easy Run 1:00:00 easy	Easy Run plus Drills and Strides 1:00:00 easy Drills and Strides	Lactate-Intervals Run 15:00 easy Drills and Strides 10 x (0:30 @ MAS/0:15 easy) 3:00 easy 10 x (0:30 @ MAS/0:15 easy) 3:00 easy 10 x (0:30 @ MAS/0:15 easy) 15:00 easy	Easy Run 1:00:00 easy	Half-Marathon Pace Run 2 miles easy Drills and Strides 2 x 3 miles @ HMP/1:00 rest 2 miles easy
11	Easy Run 30:00 easy	Tempo Run 15:00 easy Drills and Strides 18:00 @ LTP 5:00 easy 18:00 @ LTP 15:00 easy	Easy Run 1:00:00 easy	Easy Run plus Drills and Strides 1:00:00 easy Drills and Strides	Descending-Intervals Run 15:00 easy Drills and Strides 3:00 @ MAS/2:00 easy 2:00 @ MAS/1:20 easy 1:00 @ MAS/0:40 easy 0:45 @ MAS/0:30 easy 0:30 @ MAS/0:20 easy 0:45 @ MAS/0:30 easy 0:30 @ MAS/0:20 easy 15:00 easy	Easy Run 1:00:00 easy	Fast Finish Run 1:30:00 easy 10:00 @ LTP

	MONDAY	TUESDAY	WEDNESDAY	THURSDAY	FRIDAY	SATURDAY	SUNDAY
12	Rest	Progression Run 20:00 easy 16:00 @ SSP 8:00 @ LTP 4:00 @ CV 5:00 easy	Easy Run 1:00:00 easy	Easy Run plus Drills and Strides 1:00:00 easy Drills and Strides	Progression-Intervals Run 15:00 easy Drills and Strides 5 x (0:30 @ SSP/0:20 @ MAS/0:10 @ VHI) 5:00 easy 5 x (0:30 @ SSP/0:20 @ MAS/0:10 @ VHI) 5:00 easy 5 x (0:30 @ SSP/0:20 @ MAS/0:10 @ VHI) 15:00 easy	Easy Run 1:00:00 easy	Long Run 1:45:00 easy
13	Easy Run 30:00 easy	Steady-State Run 15:00 easy Drills and Strides 50:00 @ SSP 15:00 easy	Easy Run 1:00:00 easy	Easy Run plus Drills and Strides 1:00:00 easy Drills and Strides	5K Pace Intervals Run 2 miles easy Drills and Strides 8 x 600 meters @ 5KP/400 meters easy 2 miles easy	Easy Run 1:00:00 easy	Half-Marathon Pace Run 2 miles easy Drills and Strides 8 miles @ HMP 2 miles easy
14	Easy Run 30:00 easy	Over/Under Intervals Run 15:00 easy Drills and Strides 4 x (3:00 @ LTP +0:05 per mile/3:00 @ LTP -0:05 per mile/3:00 easy) 15:00 easy	Easy Run 1:00:00 easy	Easy Run plus Drills and Strides 1:00:00 easy Drills and Strides	Progression Run 30:00 easy 8:00 @ LTP 4:00 @ CV 2:00 @ MAS 5:00 easy	Easy Run 1:00:00 easy	Long Run 1:30:00 easy
15	Rest	Fartlek Run 10:00 easy 8 x 1:00 @ MAS/2:00 easy 10:00 easy	Easy Run 45:00 easy	Easy Run 45:00 easy	Fast-Finish Run 25:00 easy 10:00 @ LTP	Easy Run plus Strides 20:00 easy Drills and Strides	Half-Marathon Race

249

• LEVEL 3 •

	MONDAY	TUESDAY	WEDNESDAY	THURSDAY	FRIDAY	SATURDAY	SUNDAY
1	Easy Run 40:00 easy	Fast-Finish Run 55:00 easy 5:00 @ CV	Easy Run 45:00 easy	Easy Run plus Drills, Strides, and Plyos 1:00:00 easy Drills, Strides, and Plyos	Fartlek Run 20:00 easy Drills and Strides 10 x 0:20 @ VHI/1:20 easy 20:00 easy	Easy Run 45:00 easy	Long Run 1:20:00 easy
		Easy Run 20:00 easy			Easy Run 20:00 easy		
2	Easy Run 40:00 easy	Fast-Finish Run 50:00 easy 10:00 @ LTP	Easy Run 50:00 easy	Easy Run plus Drills, Strides, and Plyos 1:00:00 easy Drills, Strides, and Plyos	Fartlek Run 20:00 easy Drills and Strides 10 x 1:00 @ MAS/2:00 easy 20:00 easy	Easy Run 50:00 easy	Long Run 1:40:00 easy
		Easy Run 25:00 easy			Easy Run 25:00 easy		
3	Rest	Fartlek Run 20:00 easy Drills and Strides 1:00 @ 5KP 1:00 easy 2:00 @ 10KP 1:00 easy 3:00 @ HMP 1:00 easy 2:00 @ 10KP 1:00 easy 1:00 @ 5KP 1:00 easy 2:00 @ 10KP 1:00 easy 3:00 @ HMP 20:00 easy	Easy Run 45:00 easy	Easy Run plus Drills, Strides, and Plyos 1:00:00 easy Drills, Strides, and Plyos	Hill-Repetitions Run 20:00 easy Drills and Strides 10 x (0:30 uphill @ VHI/1:30 easy) 20:00 easy	Easy Run 45:00 easy	Long Run 1:30:00 easy
		Easy Run 20:00 easy			Easy Run 20:00 easy		

	MONDAY	TUESDAY	WEDNESDAY	THURSDAY	FRIDAY	SATURDAY	SUNDAY
4	Easy Run 40:00 easy	Critical-Velocity Intervals Run 20:00 easy Drills and Strides 6 x (4:00 @ CV/2:00 easy) 20:00 easy	Easy Run 55:00 easy	Easy Run plus Drills, Strides, and Plyos 1:05:00 easy Drills, Strides, and Plyos	Descending-intervals Run 20:00 easy Drills and Strides 3:00 @ MAS/2:00 easy 2:00 @ MAS/1:20 easy 1:00 @ MAS/0:40 easy 0:45 @ MAS/0:30 easy 0:30 @ MAS 20:00 easy	Easy Run 55:00 easy	Long Run 2:00:00 easy
		Easy Run 25:00 easy			Easy Run 25:00 easy		
5	Easy Run 40:00 easy	Over/Under Intervals Run 20:00 easy Drills and Strides 3 x (4:00 @ LTP plus 0:05 per mile/3:00 @ LTP-0:05 per mile/2:00 easy) 20:00 easy	Easy Run 1:00:00 easy	Easy Run plus Drills, Strides, and Plyos 1:05:00 easy Drills, Strides, and Plyos	Lactate-Intervals Run 20:00 easy Drills and Strides 10 x (0:30 @ MAS/0:15 easy) 3:00 easy 10 x (0:30 @ MAS/0:15 easy) 3:00 easy 10 x (0:30 @ MAS/0:15 easy) 20:00 easy	Easy Run 1:00:00 easy	Fast-Finish Run 1:30:00 easy 10:00 @ LTP
		Easy Run 30:00 easy			Easy Run 30:00 easy		
6	Rest	Progression Run 30:00 easy 12:00 @ SSP 6:00 @ LTP 3:00 @ CV 5:00 easy	Easy Run 55:00 easy	Easy Run plus Drills, Strides, and Plyos 1:00:00 easy Drills, Strides, and Plyos	Speed-Intervals Run 20:00 easy Drills and Strides 12 x (0:45 @ VHI/1:45 easy) 20:00 easy	Easy Run 55:00 easy	Depletion Run 1:45:00 easy, no calories before or during
		Easy Run 25:00 easy			Easy Run 25:00 easy		

(Table continues)

RUN LIKE A PRO (EVEN IF YOU'RE SLOW)

	MONDAY	TUESDAY	WEDNESDAY	THURSDAY	FRIDAY	SATURDAY	SUNDAY
7	Easy Run 40:00 easy	Steady-State Run 20:00 easy 45:00 @ SSP 20:00 easy Easy Run 30:00 easy	Easy Run 1:00:00 easy	Easy Run plus Drills, Strides, and Plyos 1:10:00 easy Drills, Strides, and Plyos Drills and Strides	Variable-Speed Intervals Run 20:00 easy Drills and Strides 5 x (4 x 0:30 @ MAS/0:45 @ LTP) 2:30 easy 20:00 easy Easy Run 30:00 easy	Easy Run 1:00:00 easy	Half-Marathon Pace Run 3 miles easy Drills and Strides 3 x 2 miles @ HMP/1:00 rest 3 miles easy
8	Easy Run 40:00 easy	Tempo Run 20:00 easy Drills and Strides 18:00 @ LTP 5:00 easy 18:00 @ LTP 20:00 easy Easy Run 35:00 easy	Easy Run 1:00:00 easy	Easy Run plus Drills, Strides, and Plyos 1:10:00 easy Drills, Strides, and Plyos	Accelerations Run 20:00 easy Drills and Strides 11:00 acceleration from jog to sprint 15:00 walk to jog 6:00 acceleration from jog to sprint 15:00 walk to jog 3:00 acceleration from jog to sprint 20:00 walk to jog Easy Run 35:00 easy	Easy Run 1:00:00 easy	Long Run 2:30:00 easy

	MONDAY	TUESDAY	WEDNESDAY	THURSDAY	FRIDAY	SATURDAY	SUNDAY
9	Rest	Fartlek Run 20:00 easy Drills and Strides 1:00 @ 5KP 1:00 easy 2:00 @ 10KP 1:00 easy 3:00 @ HMP 1:00 easy 2:00 @ 10KP 1:00 easy 1:00 @ 5KP 1:00 easy 2:00 @ 10KP 1:00 easy 3:00 @ HMP 1:00 easy 2:00 @ 10KP 1:00 easy 1:00 @ 5KP 20:00 easy Easy Run 30:00 easy	Easy Run 1:00:00 easy	Easy Run plus Drills, Strides, and Plyos 1:00:00 easy Drills, Strides, and Plyos	Hill-Repetitions Run 20:00 easy Drills and Strides 12 x (1:00 uphill @ VHI/2:00 easy) 20:00 easy Easy Run 30:00 easy	Easy Run 1:00:00 easy	Depletion Run 1:40:00 easy, no calories before or during
10	Easy Run 40:00 easy	Critical- Velocity Intervals Run 20:00 easy Drills and Strides 7 x (4:00 @ CV/2:00 easy) 20:00 easy Easy Run 35:00 easy	Easy Run 1:00:00 easy	Easy Run plus Drills, Strides, and Plyos 1:10:00 easy Drills, Strides, and Plyos	Descending- Intervals Run 20:00 easy Drills and Strides 3:00 @ MAS/2:00 easy 2:00 @ MAS/1:20 easy 1:00 @ MAS/0:40 easy 0:45 @ MAS/0:30 easy 0:30 @ MAS/0:20 easy 2:00 @ MAS/1:20 easy 1:00 @ MAS/0:40 easy 0:45 @ MAS/0:30 easy 0:30 @ MAS 20:00 easy Easy Run 35:00 easy	Easy Run 1:00:00 easy	Half- Marathon Pace Run 3 miles easy Drills and Strides 2 x 3 miles @ HMP/1:00 rest 3 miles easy

(Table continues)

	MONDAY	TUESDAY	WEDNESDAY	THURSDAY	FRIDAY	SATURDAY	SUNDAY
11	Easy Run 40:00 easy	Over/Under Intervals Run 20:00 easy Drills and Strides 4 x (3:00 @ LTP plus 0:05 per mile/3:00 @ LTP-0:05 per mile/3:00 easy) 20:00 easy Easy Run 35:00 easy	Easy Run 1:00:00 easy	Easy Run and Drills, Strides, and Plyos 1:10:00 easy Drills, Strides, and Plyos	Lactate-Intervals Run 20:00 easy Drills and Strides 12 x (0:30 @ MAS/0:15 easy) 3:00 easy 12 x (0:30 @ MAS/0:15 easy) 3:00 easy 12 x (0:30 @ MAS/0:15 easy) 20:00 easy Easy Run 35:00 easy	Easy Run 1:00:00 easy	Marathon Pace Run 2 miles easy 6 x 1 mile @ MP/1 mile easy 2 miles easy
12	Rest	Progression Run 30:00 easy 16:00 @ SSP 8:00 @ LTP 4:00 @ CV 5:00 easy Easy Run 30:00 easy	Easy Run 1:00:00 easy	Easy Run plus Drills, Strides, and Plyos 1:00:00 easy Drills, Strides, and Plyos	Progression Intervals Run 20:00 easy Drills and Strides 5 x (0:30 @ SSP/0:20 @ MAS/0:10 @ VHI) 5:00 easy 5 x (0:30 @ SSP/0:20 @ MAS/0:10 @ VHI) 5:00 easy 5 x (0:30 @ SSP/0:20 @ MAS/0:10 @ VHI) 20:00 easy Easy Run 30:00 easy	Easy Run 1:00:00 easy	Depletion Run 2:00:00 easy, no calories before or during

	MONDAY	TUESDAY	WEDNESDAY	THURSDAY	FRIDAY	SATURDAY	SUNDAY
13	Easy Run 40:00 easy	Steady-State Run 20:00 easy 55:00 @ SSP 20:00 easy Easy Run 35:00 easy	Easy Run 1:00:00 easy	Easy Run plus Drills, Strides, and Plyos 1:10:00 easy Drills, Strides, and Plyos	5K Pace Intervals Run 3 miles easy Drills and Strides 8 x 600m @ 5KP/400m easy 3 miles easy Easy Run 35:00 easy	Easy Run 1:00:00 easy	Half-Marathon Pace Run 3 miles easy Drills and Strides 8 miles @ HMP 3 miles easy
14	Easy Run 40:00 easy	10K Pace Intervals Run 3 miles easy Drills and Strides 6 x 0.75 mile @ 10KP/ 1:00 rest 3 miles easy Easy Run 30:00 easy	Easy Run 1:00:00 easy	Easy Run plus Drills, Strides, and Plyos 1:05:00 easy Drills, Strides, and Plyos	Progression Run 30:00 easy 12:00 @ LTP 6:00 @ CV 3:00 @ MAS 5:00 easy Easy Run 35:00 easy	Easy Run 1:00:00 easy	Long Run 1:40:00 easy
15	Rest	Fartlek Run 20:00 easy 10 x 1:00 @ MAS/2:00 easy 20:00 easy	Easy Run 45:00 easy	Easy Run 45:00 easy	Fast-Finish Run 30:00 easy 10:00 @ CV	Easy Run plus Strides 20:00 easy Drills and Strides	Half-Marathon Race

My Favorite
Half-Marathon Workout

> *15:00 at ten seconds slower per mile than lactate threshold pace, 8:00 jog recovery, 3 x 5:00 at ten seconds faster per mile than lactate threshold pace with 2:00 rest (5:00 after #3), 15:00 at ten seconds slower per mile than lactate threshold pace.*

The half-marathon is a tricky distance. If you try to run it off mostly marathon-specific training, you tend to lack some of the "pop" necessary to really crush it. If you try to run it off mostly 5K/10K-specific work, you lack the strength to close it down over the final few miles. And if you try to hammer workout after workout in what you consider to be the half-marathon-specific zone, then you lack a bit of the speed and strength necessary to really rock 13.1 miles. Thus, my personal theory is that in order to be at your readiest for a half marathon, you need to be coming off a block of training that is about as eclectic as you can possibly make it. It's almost like you want to accidentally be ready for a half-marathon.

I'll use one of our NAZ Elite athletes, Rory Linkletter, to explain what I mean. In January 2020, Rory ran the Aramco Houston Half Marathon in 1:01:44—the second-fastest time ever by a Canadian. Yet that race was not meant to be the culmination of his training segment. The plan, rather, was to run the half, as well as a 3K indoor track race, a 5K indoor track race, and eventually a 10K outdoor track race. That's a pretty wide range, so we hit a wide range of pace zones in his training. Over the month leading into Houston, Rory ran the following workouts:

EXAMPLE 1 (AT SEA LEVEL)

3 x 1:45 uphill (6–8 percent grade) at half-marathon effort with jog-back recoveries

3 x 0:30 uphill (6–8 percent grade) at 3K race effort with jog-back recoveries

3 x 800 meters in 2:20 with 2:00 jog recoveries

6 x 200 meters in 0:31 with 200 meter jog recoveries

5:00 rest

Three-mile tempo at 4:52/mile

EXAMPLE 2 (AT 7,000 FEET)

20 x 400 meters in 1:10 with 100-meter jog recoveries

3:00–5:00 rest

8 x 100 meters descending from 0:15 to 0:13 with 1:00 rest

EXAMPLE 3 (AT 3,100 FEET)

10 x 1K in 2:58 with 1:00 rest (5:00 rest after #10)

5K time trial in 14:21

EXAMPLE 4 (AT 7,000 FEET)

Eight-mile steady state at marathon effort (5:10 per mile)

EXAMPLE 5 (AT 3,100 FEET)

20 x 600 meters in 1:45 with 150 meter jog recoveries

3:00–5:00 rest

8 x 200 meters descending from 0:31 to 0:27 with 1:00 rest

EXAMPLE 6 (AT 7,000 FEET)

4 x 200/200/200/400 meters with 200 meter jog after the
200s, 400-meter jog between sets (200s in 0:31, 400s
in 1:02)

EXAMPLE 7 (AT 7,000 FEET)

3 miles at 5:00 per mile
3:00 rest
One mile in 4:40

As you see, I threw everything but the kitchen sink at Rory to pre-pare him for that 1:01 half-marathon. We did hills, we ran on the track, we ran on the roads, we ran slower than race pace, we ran faster than race pace, and we did a couple of things at or very near race pace.

Yet my all-time favorite half-marathon workout is one he didn't even do. The reason is that each segment is different and you have to look at context (what came before, what's coming after, etc.) when deciding which workouts are needed. In Rory's case, he was coming off a marathon segment in the fall of 2019 where he had done a ton of long, grinding sessions that were very strength-focused—similar to the one I am about to describe. And because I know such things aren't just completely out of your system simply because you take a break between segments, I felt in looking ahead to Houston that it made sense to lean toward some of the faster stuff and rely on the strength he had built while preparing for his marathon to carry him through the distance.

The results suggest I got it right that time. I don't always, of course, but it sure is nice when I do. Now, I don't know the context in which you might enter a half-marathon training segment of your own. So, I am going to take you through a session that I think is very specific to the half-marathon and would fit well into a training segment that also includes workouts geared more to the 5K and 10K and workouts geared more to the marathon.

258

For this one, you start off with a fifteen-minute tempo effort at a pace that's actually a bit slower than lactate-threshold (i.e., one-hour) pace. This is a good reminder that there's nothing magical about being smack dab in the middle of any particular training zone in a workout. In this session, I am trying to give you forty-five minutes' worth of quality volume, and that's hard to do if it's all done right at lactate-threshold pace.

Let's say your LT pace is 6:00 per mile. You'd run this first tempo at 6:10 pace—a solid effort but nothing crazy. Then I have you go straight into an eight-minute jog after the tempo. Eight minutes is probably more than necessary to recover from that sort of tempo, but it's not always about recovery. Sometimes it's about the overall volume for the entire workout. All told, including warming up and cooling down, you will end up getting nearly ninety minutes on the day. That's a heck of a lot of running. And, more important, your final few minutes of hard running will be done with nearly an hour's worth of prior running on your legs. You'll be running hard with close to the same amount of volume in your legs that you'll have as you near the end of your half-marathon.

Now on to the second section of this workout. You've done your first fifteen-minute tempo. You've jogged for eight minutes. Now you go straight into a hard five minutes at ten seconds per mile faster than your LT pace, or perhaps it's easier to say twenty seconds faster than you averaged in your tempo. So again, if you ran 6:10 pace for your fifteen-minute tempo, then you will run this five-minute effort at a 5:50 per-mile pace. Rest for two minutes by standing, walking, or jogging, and then repeat the same five-minute sequence twice more.

By this point, the workout has become very hard. When you dip under LT pace for long repeats, things get a little crazy. You're tired. You hit the five-minute repeats, but you think there's absolutely no way you are going to be able to run the final fifteen-minute tempo. You take five full minutes to walk around, sip on your electrolyte drink, think negative thoughts, and wonder what kind of sadist would come up with such a workout, and then off you go. (At least, that's

259

what I have witnessed in the NAZ Elite athletes when they're given this workout.)

But then, something amazing happens. You get out and find 6:10 pace and it's not as bad as you thought. You're doing it. The negative thoughts change to positive ones. You begin to realize this thing is doable. You get to the ten-minute mark and you are spot-on. Now you're almost, dare I say, enjoying this final stretch. You finish and you are a little bit surprised, sure, but mostly you are just pretty darn proud of yourself. And that's a nice way to finish a hard workout.

MARATHON TRAINING PLANS

T HE MARATHON HAS A mystique that no other running event can match. This special allure comes partly from the rich history of the event, which extends all the way back to ancient Greece. But it also comes from the unique challenge that the distance presents. Most marathon veterans would agree that 26.2 miles is just slightly too far to truly race, yet it's somehow raceable—if you prepare correctly.

One of the advantages of the fact that the marathon has been around as long as it has is that the top professionals and their coaches have figured out how to prepare for it correctly. The three training plans offered in this chapter represent pro-style marathon preparation. The level 1 plan features four runs per week, plus two sessions that may be done either as easy runs or as nonimpact cardio cross-training sessions, and a rest day. You should be able to run comfortably for at least an hour before you begin this plan. The level 2 plan features seven runs per week (six in recovery weeks), and you should be running daily for up to eighty minutes before you begin. Finally, the level 3 plan features nine runs per week (eight in recovery weeks), and you should have a solid fitness base that includes daily running and some work at higher intensities before you start it.

All three plans contain three-week step cycles, where the training load is reduced for recovery in the third week. Refer back to the Training Plans Overview for details on how to do the various workout types. Coach Ben's favorite marathon workout is described in a pro tip that follows this chapter. Interactive, online versions of these training plans—plus a beginner-friendly level 0 plan—are available at 8020endurance.com. Adaptive versions are available through the PACE smartphone app.

· LEVEL 1 ·

	MONDAY	TUESDAY	WEDNESDAY	THURSDAY	FRIDAY	SATURDAY	SUNDAY
1	Rest	Fast Finish Run 35:00 easy 5:00 @ CV	Easy Run or Cross-Training 30:00 easy	Easy Run 30:00 easy	Fartlek Run 10:00 easy Drills and Strides 6 x 0:20 @ VHI/1:20 easy 10:00 easy	Easy Run or Cross-Training 30:00 easy	Long Run 7 miles easy
2	Rest	Fast-Finish Run 35:00 easy 10:00 @ LTP	Easy Run or Cross-Training 35:00 easy	Easy Run 35:00 easy	Fartlek Run 10:00 easy Drills and Strides 6 x 1:00 @ MAS/2:00 easy 10:00 easy	Easy Run or Cross-Training 35:00 easy	Long Run 8 miles easy
3	Rest	Fartlek Run 10:00 easy 1:00 @ 5KP 1:00 easy 2:00 @ 10KP 1:00 easy 3:00 @ HMP 1:00 easy 2:00 @ 10KP 1:00 easy 1:00 @ 5KP 10:00 easy	Easy Run or Cross-Training 30:00 easy	Easy Run 30:00 easy	Hill-Repetitions Run 10:00 easy Drills and Strides 6 x (0:30 uphill @ VHI/1:30 easy) 10:00 easy	Easy Run or Cross-Training 30:00 easy	Long Run 7 miles easy
4	Rest	Critical-Velocity Intervals Run 10:00 easy Drills and Strides 4 x (4:00 @ CV/2:00 easy) 10:00 easy	Easy Run or Cross-Training 35:00 easy	Easy Run 40:00 easy	Fartlek Run 10:00 easy Drills and Strides 8 x 1:00 @ MAS/2:00 easy 10:00 easy	Easy Run or Cross-Training 35:00 easy	Long Run 9 miles easy

	MONDAY	TUESDAY	WEDNESDAY	THURSDAY	FRIDAY	SATURDAY	SUNDAY
5	Rest	Over/Under Intervals Run 10:00 easy Drills and Strides 3 x (3:00 @ LTP +0:05 per mile/3:00 @ LTP -0:05 per mile/3:00 easy) 10:00 easy	Easy Run or Cross-Training 40:00 easy	Easy Run 45:00 easy	5K Pace Intervals Run 1 mile easy Drills and Strides 6 x 800 meters @ 5KP/1:00 rest 1 mile easy	Easy Run or Cross-Training 40:00 easy	Long Run 10 miles easy
6	Rest	Progression Run 30:00 easy 8:00 @ SSP 4:00 @ LTP 2:00 @ CV 5:00 easy	Easy Run or Cross-Training 35:00 easy	Easy Run 35:00 easy	Speed-Intervals Run 10:00 easy Drills and Strides 8 x 0:45 @ VHI/1:45 walk-to-jog 10:00 easy	Easy Run or Cross-Training 35:00 easy	Long Run 8 miles easy
7	Rest	Steady-State Run 10:00 easy Drills and Strides 30:00 @ SSP 10:00 easy	Easy Run or Cross-Training 40:00 easy	Easy Run 50:00 easy	Progression Run 30:00 easy 8:00 @ LTP 4:00 @ CV 2:00 @ MAS 5:00 easy	Easy Run or Cross-Training 40:00 easy	Long Run 11 miles easy
8	Rest	Critical-Velocity Intervals Run 10:00 easy Drills and Strides 5 x (4:00 @ CV/2:00 easy) 10:00 easy	Easy Run or Cross-Training 45:00 easy	Easy Run 55:00 easy	Descending-Intervals Run 10:00 easy Drills and Strides 3:00 @ MAS/2:00 easy 2:00 @ MAS/1:20 easy 1:00 @ MAS/0:40 easy 0:45 @ MAS/0:30 easy 0:30 @ MAS 10:00 easy	Easy Run or Cross-Training 45:00 easy	Long Run 12 miles easy

(Table continues)

RUN LIKE A PRO (EVEN IF YOU'RE SLOW)

	MONDAY	TUESDAY	WEDNESDAY	THURSDAY	FRIDAY	SATURDAY	SUNDAY
9	Rest	Fartlek Run 10:00 easy Drills and Strides 1:00 @ 5KP 1:00 easy 2:00 @ 10KP 1:00 easy 3:00 @ HMP 1:00 easy 2:00 @ 10KP 1:00 easy 1:00 @ 5KP 1:00 easy 2:00 @ 10KP 1:00 easy 3:00 @ HMP 10:00 easy	Easy Run or Cross-Training 40:00 easy	Easy Run 40:00 easy	Hill-Repetitions Run 10:00 easy Drills and Strides 6 x (1:00 uphill @ VHI/2:00 easy) 10:00 easy	Easy Run or Cross-Training 40:00 easy	Long Run 9 miles easy
10	Rest	Tempo Run 10:00 easy Drills and Strides 12:00 @ LTP 5:00 easy 12:00 @ LTP 10:00 easy	Easy Run or Cross-Training 45:00 easy	Easy Run 1:00:00 easy	Variable-Speed Intervals Run 10:00 easy Drills and Strides 3 x (4 x 0:30 @ MAS/0:45 @ LTP) 2:30 easy 10:00 easy	Easy Run or Cross-Training 45:00 easy	Long Run 13 miles easy
11	Rest	Steady-State Run 10:00 easy Drills and Strides 35:00 @ SSP 10:00 easy	Easy Run or Cross-Training 50:00 easy	Easy Run 1:00:00 easy	Accelerations Run 10:00 easy Drills and Strides 11:00 acceleration from jog to sprint 10:00 walk to jog 3:00 acceleration from jog to sprint 10:00 walk to jog	Easy Run or Cross-Training 50:00 easy	Long Run 14 miles easy

	MONDAY	TUESDAY	WEDNESDAY	THURSDAY	FRIDAY	SATURDAY	SUNDAY
12	Rest	Progression Run 20:00 easy 12:00 @ SSP 6:00 @ LTP 3:00 @ CV 5:00 easy	Easy Run or Cross-Training 45:00 easy	Easy Run 45:00 easy	Speed-Intervals Run 10:00 easy Drills and Strides 8 x 1:00 @ VHI/2:00 walk to jog 10:00 easy	Easy Run or Cross-Training 45:00 easy	Long Run 10 miles easy
13	Rest	10K Pace Intervals Run 1 mile easy Drills and Strides 8 x 1 kilometer @ 10KP/ 1:00 rest 1 mile easy	Easy Run or Cross-Training 50:00 easy	Easy Run 1:00:00 easy	Lactate-Intervals run 10:00 easy Drills and Strides 8 x (0:30 @ MAS/0:15 easy) 3:00 easy 8 x (0:30 @ MAS/0:15 easy) 3:00 easy 8 x (0:30 @ MAS/0:15 easy) 10:00 easy	Easy Run or Cross-Training 50:00 easy	Long Run 16 miles easy
14	Rest	Over/Under Intervals Run 10:00 easy Drills and Strides 3 x (3:00 @ LTP plus 0:05 per mile/4:00 @ LTP-0:05 per mile/2:00 easy) 10:00 easy	Easy Run or Cross-Training 55:00 easy	Easy Run 1:00:00 easy	Progression Intervals Run 10:00 easy Drills and Strides 5 x (0:30 @ SSP/0:20 @ MAS/0:10 @ VHI) 5:00 easy 5 x (0:30 @ SSP/0:20 @ MAS/0:10 @ VHI) 10:00 easy	Easy Run or Cross-Training 55:00 easy	Long Run 18 miles easy

(Table continues)

	MONDAY	TUESDAY	WEDNESDAY	THURSDAY	FRIDAY	SATURDAY	SUNDAY
15	Rest	Fartlek Run 10:00 easy Drills and Strides 1:00 @ 5KP 1:00 easy 2:00 @ 10KP 1:00 easy 3:00 @ HMP 1:00 easy 2:00 @ 10KP 1:00 easy 1:00 @ 5KP 1:00 easy 2:00 @ 10KP 1:00 easy 3:00 @ HMP 10:00 easy	Easy Run or Cross-Training 45:00 easy	Easy Run 45:00 easy	Hill Repetitions Run 10:00 easy Drills and Strides 4 x (2:00 uphill @ HI/3:00 easy) 10:00 easy	Easy Run or Cross-Training 45:00 easy	Long Run 12 miles easy
16	Rest	Relaxed 10K Time Trial 1 mile easy Drills and Strides 10KP @ 10KP plus 5 percent 1 mile easy	Easy Run or Cross-Training 1:00:00 easy	Easy Run 1:00:00 easy	5K Pace Intervals Run 1 mile easy Drills and Strides 8 x 600 meters @ 5KP/1:00 rest 1 mile easy	Easy Run or Cross-Training 1:00:00 easy	Coach Ben's Favorite Marathon Workout 10:00 easy 1:00:00 @ SSP plus 1:00/ mile 1:00 @ SSP 10:00 easy
17	Rest	Tempo Run 10:00 easy Drills and Strides 14:00 @ LTP 5:00 easy 14:00 @ LTP 10:00 easy	Easy Run or Cross-Training 1:00:00 easy	Easy Run 55:00 easy	Progression Run 30:00 easy 8:00 @ LTP 4:00 @ CV 2:00 @ MAS 5:00 easy	Easy Run or Cross-Training 50:00 easy	Long Run 10 miles easy
18	Rest	Fartlek Run 10:00 easy Drills and Strides 5 x 1:00 @ MAS/2:00 easy 10:00 easy	Easy Run or Cross-Training 40:00 easy	Easy Run 35:00 easy	Fast-Finish Run 25:00 easy 10:00 @ LTP	Easy Run plus Strides 20:00 easy Drills and Strides	Marathon Race

· LEVEL 2 ·

	MONDAY	TUESDAY	WEDNESDAY	THURSDAY	FRIDAY	SATURDAY	SUNDAY
1	Easy Run 30:00 easy	Fast-Finish Run 40:00 easy 10:00 @ LTP	Easy Run 45:00 easy	Easy Run plus Drills and Strides 45:00 easy Drills and Strides	Fartlek Run 15:00 easy Drills and Strides 8 x 0:20 @ VHI/1:20 easy 15:00 easy	Easy Run 45:00 easy	Long Run 10 miles easy
2	Easy Run 30:00 easy	Fast-Finish Run 45:00 easy 5:00 @ CV	Easy Run 45:00 easy	Easy Run plus Drills and Strides 45:00 easy Drills and Strides	Fartlek Run 15:00 easy Drills and Strides 8 x 1:00 @ MAS/2:00 easy 15:00 easy	Easy Run 45:00 easy	Long Run 12 miles easy
3	Rest	Fartlek Run 15:00 easy Drills and Strides 1:00 @ 5KP 1:00 easy 2:00 @ 10KP 1:00 easy 3:00 @ HMP 1:00 easy 2:00 @ 10KP 1:00 easy 1:00 @ 5KP 1:00 easy 2:00 @ 10KP 1:00 easy 3:00 @ HMP 15:00 easy	Easy Run 45:00 easy	Easy Run plus Drills and Strides 45:00 easy Drills and Strides	Hill-Repetitions Run 15:00 easy Drills and Strides 8 x (0:30 uphill @ VHI/1:30 easy) 15:00 easy	Easy Run 45:00 easy	Long Run 10 miles easy
4	Easy Run 30:00 easy	Critical-Velocity Intervals Run 15:00 easy Drills and Strides 5 x (4:00 @ CV/2:00 easy) 15:00 easy	Easy Run 50:00 easy	Easy Run plus Drills and Strides 50:00 easy Drills and Strides	Fartlek Run 15:00 easy Drills and Strides 10 x 1:00 @ MAS/2:00 easy 15:00 easy	Easy Run 50:00 easy	Long Run 14 miles easy

(Table continues)

267

RUN LIKE A PRO (EVEN IF YOU'RE SLOW)

	MONDAY	TUESDAY	WEDNESDAY	THURSDAY	FRIDAY	SATURDAY	SUNDAY
5	Easy Run 30:00 easy	Over/Under Intervals Run 15:00 easy Drills and Strides 3 x (3:00 @ LTP +0:05 per mile/4:00 @ LTP -0:05 per mile/2:00 easy) 15:00 easy	Easy Run 50:00 easy	Easy Run plus Drills and Strides 50:00 easy Drills and Strides	5K Pace Intervals Run 2 miles easy Drills and Strides 6 x 800m @ 5KP/400m easy 2 miles easy	Easy Run 50:00 easy	Long Run 17 miles easy
6	Rest	Progression Run 30:00 easy 12:00 @ SSP 6:00 @ LTP 3:00 @ CV 5:00 easy	Easy Run 45:00 easy	Easy Run plus Drills and Strides 45:00 easy Drills and Strides	Leg-Speed Run 15:00 easy Drills and Strides 10 x 0:45 @ VHI/1:45 walk to jog 15:00 easy 30-20-10 Run 15:00 easy Drills and Strides 5 x (0:30 @ SSP/0:20 @ MAS/0:10 @ VHI) 5:00 easy 5 x (0:30 @ SSP/0:20 @ MAS/0:10 @ VHI) 5:00 easy 5 x (0:30 @ SSP/0:20 @ MAS/0:10 @ VHI) 15:00 easy	Easy Run 45:00 easy	Long Run 12 miles easy
7	Easy Run 30:00 easy	Steady-State Run 15:00 easy 35:00 @ SSP 15:00 easy	Easy Run 55:00 easy	Easy Run plus Drills and Strides 55:00 easy Drills and Strides	Descending-Intervals Run 15:00 easy Drills and Strides 3:00 @ MAS/2:00 easy 2:00 @ MAS/1:20 easy 1:00 @ MAS/0:40 easy 0:45 @ MAS/0:30 easy 0:30 @ MAS/0:20 easy 0:45 @ MAS/0:30 easy 0:30 @ MAS/ 15:00 easy	Easy Run 55:00 easy	Depletion Run 14 miles easy, no calories before or during

	MONDAY	TUESDAY	WEDNESDAY	THURSDAY	FRIDAY	SATURDAY	SUNDAY
8	Easy Run 30:00 easy	10K Pace Intervals Run 2 miles easy Drills and Strides 8 x 1 kilometer @ 10KP/ 1:00 rest 2 miles easy	Easy Run 55:00 easy	Easy Run plus Drills and Strides 55:00 easy Drills and Strides	Progression Run 30:00 easy 12:00 @ LTP 6:00 @ CV 3:00 @ MAS 5:00 easy	Easy Run 55:00 easy	Marathon Pace Run 1 mile easy Drills and Strides 7 x 1 mile easy/1 mile @ MP 1 mile easy
9	Rest	Fartlek Run 15:00 easy Drills and Strides 1:00 @ 5KP 1:00 easy 2:00 @ 10KP 1:00 easy 3:00 @ HMP 1:00 easy 2:00 @ 10KP 1:00 easy 1:00 @ 5KP 1:00 easy 2:00 @ 10KP 1:00 easy 3:00 @ HMP 1:00 easy 2:00 @ 10KP 1:00 easy 1:00 @ 5KP 15:00 easy	Easy Run 50:00 easy	Easy Run plus Drills and Strides 50:00 easy Drills and Strides	Hill-Repetitions Run 15:00 easy Drills and Strides 8 x (1:00 uphill @ Hi/2:00 easy) 15:00 easy	Easy Run 50:00 easy	Long Run with Fast Finish 12 miles easy 2 miles @ HMP
10	Easy Run 30:00 easy	Tempo Run 15:00 easy Drills and Strides 16:00 @ LTP 5:00 easy 16:00 @ LTP 15:00 easy	Easy Run 1:00:00 easy	Easy Run plus Drills and Strides 1:00:00 easy Drills and Strides	Variable-Speed Intervals Run 15:00 easy Drills and Strides 4 x (4 x 0:30 @ MAS/0:45 @ LTP) 2:30 easy 15:00 easy	Easy Run 1:00:00 easy	Long Run 20 miles easy

(Table continues)

	MONDAY	TUESDAY	WEDNESDAY	THURSDAY	FRIDAY	SATURDAY	SUNDAY
11	Easy Run 30:00 easy	Steady-State Run 15:00 easy Drills and Strides 40:00 @ SSP 15:00 easy	Easy Run 1:00:00 easy	Easy Run plus Drills and Strides 1:00:00 easy Drills and Strides	Accelerations Run 15:00 easy Drills and Strides 11:00 acceleration from jog to sprint 10:00 walk to jog 6:00 acceleration from jog to sprint 15:00 walk to jog	Easy Run 1:00:00 easy	Marathon Pace Run 2 miles easy Drills and Strides 12 miles @ MP 2 miles easy
12	Rest	Progression Run 30:00 easy 16:00 @ SSP 8:00 @ LTP 4:00 @ CV 5:00 easy	Easy Run 50:00 easy	Easy Run plus Drills and Strides 50:00 easy Drills and Strides	Leg-Speed Run 15:00 easy Drills and Strides 10 x 1:00 @ VHI/2:00 walk to jog 15:00 easy	Easy Run 50:00 easy	Depletion Run 16 miles easy, no calories before or during
13	Easy Run 30:00 easy	Critical-Velocity Intervals Run 15:00 easy Drills and Strides 6 x (4:00 @ CV/2:00 easy) 15:00 easy	Easy Run 1:00:00 easy	Easy Run plus Drills and Strides 1:05:00 easy Drills and Strides	Lactate-Intervals Run 15:00 easy Drills and Strides 10 x (0:30 @ MAS/0:15 easy) 3:00 easy 10 x (0:30 @ MAS/0:15 easy) 3:00 easy 10 x (0:30 @ MAS/0:15 easy) 15:00 easy	Easy Run 1:00:00 easy	Long Run 22 miles easy
14	Easy Run 30:00 easy	Over/Under Intervals Run 15:00 easy Drills and Strides 4 x (3:00 @ LTP plus 0:05 per mile/3:00 @ LTP-0:05 per mile/3:00 easy) 15:00 easy	Easy Run 1:00:00 easy	Easy Run plus Drills and Strides 1:05:00 easy Drills and Strides	Progression Intervals Run 15:00 easy Drills and Strides 5 x (0:30 @ SSP/0:20 @ MAS/0:10 @ VHI) 5:00 easy 5 x (0:30 @ SSP/0:20 @ MAS/0:10 @ VHI) 15:00 easy	Easy Run 1:00:00 easy	Marathon Pace Run 2 miles easy Drills and Strides 15 miles @ MP 2 miles easy

	MONDAY	TUESDAY	WEDNESDAY	THURSDAY	FRIDAY	SATURDAY	SUNDAY
15	Rest	Fartlek Run 15:00 easy Drills and Strides 1:00 @ 5KP 1:00 easy 2:00 @ 10KP 1:00 easy 3:00 @ HMP 1:00 easy 2:00 @ 10KP 1:00 easy 1:00 @ 5KP 1:00 easy 2:00 @ 10KP 1:00 easy 3:00 @ HMP 1:00 easy 2:00 @ 10KP 1:00 easy 1:00 @ 5KP 15:00 easy	Easy Run 50:00 easy	Easy Run plus Drills and Strides 55:00 easy Drills and Strides	Hill-Repetitions Run 15:00 easy Drills and Strides 5 x (2:00 uphill @ VHI/3:00 easy) 15:00 easy	Easy Run 50:00 easy	Long Run 12 miles easy
16	Easy Run 30:00 easy	Relaxed 10K Time Trial 2 miles easy Drills and Strides 10KP @ 10KP + 5% 2 miles easy	Easy Run 1:00:00 easy	Easy Run plus Drills and Strides 1:10:00 easy Drills and Strides	5K Pace Intervals Run 2 miles easy Drills and Strides 8 x 600 meters @ 5KP/400 meters easy 2 miles easy	Easy Run 1:00:00 easy	Coach Ben's Favorite Marathon Workout 15:00 easy 1:00:00 @ SSP plus 1:00/mile 1:00 @ SSP 15:00 easy
17	Easy Run 30:00 easy	Tempo Run 15:00 easy Drills and Strides 20:00 @ LTP 5:00 easy 20:00 @ LTP 15:00 easy	Easy Run 1:00:00 easy	Easy Run plus Drills and Strides 55:00 easy Drills and Strides	Progression Run 30:00 easy 12:00 @ LTP 6:00 @ CV 3:00 @ MAS 5:00 easy	Easy Run 50:00 easy	Long Run 12 miles easy
18	Rest	Fartlek Run 15:00 easy Drills and Strides 8 x 1:00 @ MAS/2:00 easy 15:00 easy	Easy Run 45:00 easy	Fast-Finish Run 35:00 easy 10:00 @ LTP	Easy Run 40:00 easy	Easy Run plus Strides 20:00 easy Drills and Strides	Marathon Race

271

	MONDAY	TUESDAY	WEDNESDAY	THURSDAY	FRIDAY	SATURDAY	SUNDAY
1	Easy Run 40:00 easy	Fast-Finish Run 55:00 easy 5:00 @ CV Easy Run 20:00 easy	Easy Run 1:00:00 easy	Easy Run plus Drills, Strides, and Plyos 1:00:00 easy Drills, Strides, and Plyos	Fartlek Run 20:00 easy Drills and Strides 10 x 0:20 @ VHI/1:20 easy 20:00 easy Easy Run 20:00 easy	Easy Run 1:00:00 easy	Long Run 14 miles easy
2	Easy Run 40:00 easy	Fast-Finish Run 50:00 easy 10:00 @ LTP Easy Run 25:00 easy	Easy Run 1:00:00 easy	Easy Run plus Drills, Strides, and Plyos 1:00:00 easy Drills, Strides, and Plyos	Fartlek Run 20:00 easy Drills and Strides 10 x 1:00 @ MAS/2:00 easy 20:00 easy Easy Run 25:00 easy	Easy Run 1:00:00 easy	Long Run 16 miles easy
3	Rest	Fartlek Run 20:00 easy Drills and Strides 1:00 @ 5KP 1:00 easy 2:00 @ 10KP 1:00 easy 5:00 @ HMP 1:00 easy 2:00 @ 10KP 1:00 easy 1:00 @ 5KP 1:00 easy 2:00 @ 10KP 1:00 easy 5:00 @ HMP 20:00 easy Easy Run 20:00 easy	Easy Run 1:00:00 easy	Easy Run plus Drills, Strides, and Plyos 1:00:00 easy Drills, Strides, and Plyos	Hill Repetitions Run 20:00 easy Drills and Strides 10 x (0:30 uphill @ VHI/1:30 easy) 20:00 easy Easy Run 20:00 easy	Easy Run 1:00:00 easy	Depletion Run 1:40:00 easy, no calories before or during

	MONDAY	TUESDAY	WEDNESDAY	THURSDAY	FRIDAY	SATURDAY	SUNDAY
4	Easy Run 40:00 easy	Critical-Velocity Intervals Run 20:00 easy Drills and Strides 6 x (4:00 @ CV/2:00 easy) 20:00 easy	Easy Run 1:00:00 easy	Easy Run plus Drills, Strides, and Plyos 1:05:00 easy Drills, Strides, and Plyos	Lactate-Intervals run 20:00 easy Drills and Strides 10 x (0:30 @ MAS/0:15 easy) 3:00 easy 10 x (0:30 @ MAS/0:15 easy) 3:00 easy 10 x (0:30 @ MAS/0:15 easy) 20:00 easy	Easy Run 1:00:00 easy	Long Run 18 miles easy
		Easy Run 25:00 easy			Easy Run 25:00 easy		
5	Easy Run 40:00 easy	Tempo Run 20:00 easy Drills and Strides 16:00 @ LTP 5:00 easy 16:00 @ LTP 20:00 easy	Easy Run 1:00:00 easy	Easy Run plus Drills, Strides, and Plyos 1:05:00 easy Drills, Strides, and Plyos	5K Pace Intervals Run 3 miles easy Drills and Strides 6 x 800 meters @ 5KP/1:00 rest 3 miles easy	Easy Run 1:00:00 easy	Half-Marathon Pace Run 3 miles easy Drills and Strides 3 x 2 miles @ HMP/1:00 rest 3 miles easy
		Easy Run 30:00 easy			Easy Run 30:00 easy		
6	Rest	Progression Run 40:00 easy 12:00 @ SSP 6:00 @ LTP 3:00 @ CV 5:00 easy	Easy Run 1:00:00 easy	Easy Run plus Drills, Strides, and Plyos 1:00:00 easy Drills, Strides, and Plyos	Speed-Intervals Run 20:00 easy Drills and Strides 12 x 0:45 @ VHI/1:45 walk to jog 20:00 easy	Easy Run 1:00:00 easy	Long Run with Fast Finish 1:30:00 easy 10:00 @ LTP
		Easy Run 25:00 easy			Easy Run 25:00 easy		

(Table continues)

273

	MONDAY	TUESDAY	WEDNESDAY	THURSDAY	FRIDAY	SATURDAY	SUNDAY
7	Easy Run 40:00 easy	10K Pace Intervals Run 3 miles easy Drills and Strides 10 x 1 km @ 10KP/ 1:00 rest 3 miles easy	Easy Run 1:00:00 easy	Easy Run plus Drills, Strides, and Plyos 1:10:00 easy Drills, Strides, and Plyos	Descending Intervals Run 20:00 easy Drills and Strides 3:00 @ MAS/2:00 easy 2:00 @ MAS/1:20 easy 1:00 @ MAS/0:40 easy 0:45 @ MAS/0:30 easy 0:30 @ MAS/0:20 easy 2:00 @ MAS/1:20 easy 1:00 @ MAS/0:40 easy 0:45 @ MAS/0:30 easy 0:30 @ MAS 20:00 easy	Easy Run 1:00:00 easy	Marathon Pace Run 1 mile easy Drills and Strides 7 x 1 mile easy/1 mile @ MP 1 mile easy
		Easy Run 30:00 easy			Easy Run 30:00 easy		
8	Easy Run 40:00 easy	Tempo Run 20:00 easy Drills and Stride 18:00 @ LTP 5:00 easy 18:00 @ LTP 20:00 easy	Easy Run 1:00:00 easy	Easy Run plus Drills, Strides, and Plyos 1:10:00 easy Drills, Strides, and Plyos	Progression Run 40:00 easy 12:00 @ LTP 6:00 @ CV 3:00 @ MAS 5:00 easy	Easy Run 1:00:00 easy	Long Run 20 miles easy
		Easy Run 35:00 easy			Easy Run 35:00 easy		

	MONDAY	TUESDAY	WEDNESDAY	THURSDAY	FRIDAY	SATURDAY	SUNDAY
9	Rest	Fartlek Run 20:00 easy Drills and Strides 1:00 @ 5KP 1:00 easy 2:00 @ 10KP 1:00 easy 5:00 @ HMP 1:00 easy 2:00 @ 10KP 1:00 easy 1:00 @ 5KP 1:00 easy 2:00 @ 10KP 1:00 easy 5:00 @ HMP 1:00 easy 2:00 @ 10KP 1:00 easy 1:00 @ 10KP 20:00 easy Easy Run 30:00 easy	Easy Run 1:00:00 easy	Easy Run plus Drills, Strides, and Plyos 1:00:00 easy Drills, Strides, and Plyos	Hill-Repetitions Run 20:00 easy Drills and Strides 12 x (1:00 uphill @ VHI/2:00 easy) 20:00 easy Easy Run 30:00 easy	Easy Run 1:00:00 easy	Depletion Run 2:00:00 easy, no calories before or during
10	Easy Run 40:00 easy	Steady-State Run 20:00 easy Drills and Strides 50:00 @ SSP 20:00 easy Easy Run 35:00 easy	Easy Run 1:00:00 easy	Easy Run plus Drills, Strides, and Plyos 1:15:00 easy Drills, Strides, and Plyos	Accelerations Run 20:00 easy Drills and Strides 11:00 acceleration from jog to sprint 10:00 walk to jog 6:00 acceleration from jog to sprint 10:00 walk to jog 3:00 acceleration from jog to sprint 20:00 walk to jog Easy Run 35:00 easy	Easy Run 1:00:00 easy	Marathon Pace Run 2 miles easy 12 miles @ MP 2 miles easy

(Table continues)

	MONDAY	TUESDAY	WEDNESDAY	THURSDAY	FRIDAY	SATURDAY	SUNDAY
11	Easy Run 40:00 easy	Critical-Velocity Intervals Run 20:00 easy Drills and Strides 7 x (4:00 @ CV/2:00 easy) 20:00 easy Easy Run 35:00 easy	Easy Run 1:00:00 easy	Easy Run plus Drills, Strides, and Plyos 1:15:00 easy Drills, Strides, and Plyos	Variable-Speed Intervals Run 20:00 easy Drills and Strides 5 x (4 x 0:30 @ MAS/0:45 @ LTP) 2:30 easy 20:00 easy Easy Run 35:00 easy	Easy Run 1:00:00 easy	Long Run 24 miles easy
12	Rest	Progression Run 40:00 easy 16:00 @ SSP 8:00 @ LTP 4:00 @ CV 5:00 easy Easy Run 30:00 easy	Easy Run 1:00:00 easy	Easy Run plus Drills, Strides, and Plyos 1:15:00 easy Drills, Strides, and Plyos	Speed-Intervals Run 20:00 easy Drills and Strides 12 x 1:00 @ VHI/2:00 walk to jog 20:00 easy Easy Run 30:00 easy	Easy Run 1:00:00 easy	Long Run with Fast Finish 1:40:00 easy 10:00 @ LTP
13	Easy Run 40:00 easy	10K Pace Run 3 miles easy Drills and Strides 8 x 1 kilometer @ 10KP/1:00 rest 3 miles easy Easy Run 35:00 easy	Easy Run 1:00:00 easy	Easy Run + Drills, Strides, and Plyos 1:15:00 easy Drills, Strides, and Plyos	Lactate Intervals run 20:00 easy Drills and Strides 12 x (0:30 @ MAS/0:15 easy) 3:00 easy 12 x (0:30 @ MAS/0:15 easy) 3:00 easy 12 x (0:30 @ MAS/0:15 easy) 20:00 easy Easy Run 35:00 easy	Easy Run 1:00:00 easy	Marathon Pace Run 2 miles easy Drills and Strides 12 miles @ MP 2 miles easy

	MONDAY	TUESDAY	WEDNESDAY	THURSDAY	FRIDAY	SATURDAY	SUNDAY
14	Easy Run 40:00 easy	Over/Under Intervals Run 20:00 easy Drills and Strides 4 x (4:00 @ LTP plus 0:05 per mile/3:00 @ LTP-0:05 per mile/2:00 easy) 20:00 easy	Easy Run 1:00:00 easy	Easy Run plus Drills, Strides, and Plyos 1:15:00 easy Drills, Strides, and Plyos	Progression Intervals Run 20:00 easy Drills and Strides 5 x (0:30 @ SSP/0:20 @ MAS/0:10 @ VHI) 5:00 easy 5 x (0:30 @ SSP/0:20 @ MAS/0:10 @ VHI) 5:00 easy 5 x (0:30 @ SSP/0:20 @ MAS/0:10 @ VHI) 5:00 easy 5 x (0:30 @ SSP/0:20 @ MAS/0:10 @ VHI) 20:00 easy	Easy Run 1:00:00 easy	Half-Marathon Pace Run 2 miles easy Drills and Strides 2 x 3 miles @ HMP/1:00 rest 2 miles easy
		Easy Run 35:00 easy			Easy Run 35:00 easy		
15	Rest	Fartlek Run 20:00 easy Drills and Strides 1:00 @ 5KP 1:00 easy 2:00 @ 10KP 1:00 easy 5:00 @ HMP 1:00 easy 2:00 @ 10KP 1:00 easy 1:00 @ 5KP 1:00 easy 2:00 @ 10KP 1:00 easy 5:00 @ HMP 1:00 easy 2:00 @ 10KP 1:00 easy 1:00 @ 10KP 20:00 easy	Easy Run 1:00:00 easy	Easy Run plus Drills, Strides, and Plyos 1:15:00 easy Drills, Strides, and Plyos	Hill-Repetitions Run 20:00 easy Drills and Strides 6 x (2:00 uphill @ VHI/3:00 easy) 20:00 easy	Easy Run 1:00:00 easy	Depletion Run 2:20:00 easy, no calories before or during
		Easy Run 30:00 easy			Easy Run 30:00 easy		

(Table continues) 277

	MONDAY	TUESDAY	WEDNESDAY	THURSDAY	FRIDAY	SATURDAY	SUNDAY
16	Easy Run 40:00 easy	Relaxed 10K Time Trial 3 miles easy Drills and Strides 10KP @ 10KP plus 5 percent 3 miles easy Easy Run 35:00 easy	Easy Run 1:00:00 easy	Easy Run plus Drills, Strides, and Plyos 1:15:00 easy Drills, Strides, and Plyos	5K Pace Intervals Run 3 miles easy Drills and Strides 8 x 600 meters @ 5KP/1:00 rest 3 miles easy Easy Run 35:00 easy	Easy Run 1:00:00 easy	Coach Ben's Favorite Marathon Workout 20:00 easy 1:00:00 @ SSP plus 1:00/mile 1:00 @ SSP 20:00 easy
17	Easy Run 40:00 easy	Tempo Run 20:00 easy Drills and Stride 22:00 @ LTP 5:00 easy 22:00 @ LTP 20:00 easy Easy Run 30:00 easy	Easy Run 1:00:00 easy	Easy Run plus Drills and Strides 1:00:00 easy Drills and Strides	Progression Run 40:00 easy 12:00 @ LTP 6:00 @ CV 3:00 @ MAS 5:00 easy Easy Run 30:00 easy	Easy Run 1:00:00 easy	Long Run 14 miles easy
18	Rest	Marathon Pace Run 3 miles easy Drills and Strides 6 miles @ MP 3 miles easy	Easy Run 1:00:00 easy	Fartlek Run 20:00 easy Drills and Strides 8 x 1:00 @ MAS/2:00 easy 20:00 easy	Easy Run 40:00 easy	Easy Run plus Strides 20:00 easy Drills and Strides	Marathon Race

Coach's Tip

My Favorite
Marathon Workout

Two hours continuous running with the first hour at
steady state pace plus fifty seconds per mile and the
second hour at steady state pace

In the last chapter, I called the half-marathon a tricky distance to coach. In contrast, I actually find the marathon to be the easiest event to coach—at least in terms of the nuts and bolts. The reason is that, in the marathon, the pace is not really the issue. Let's say you're someone for whom it would be realistic to run 7:00 per mile for the marathon. For you, then, seven minutes is not a fast mile. It doesn't spike your heart rate or cause you to breathe hard. You could probably go out most days and run for a good long while at this pace without much trouble. But can your muscles and tendons and ligaments handle the pounding of twenty-six straight miles on the pavement at seven minutes per mile without breaking down? This is the million dollar question in marathon training.

In my experience with the pros, ensuring an affirmative answer requires a training process that includes lots of workouts over an eight- to ten-week period leading into the race that are made up of ten to sixteen miles of work at or near race pace, on pavement, on fairly tired legs—courtesy of high overall weekly volume. That's not to say every single workout is of this variety. I do incorporate occasional sessions that are a little faster for the sake of variety and efficiency, but at least once a week—and usually twice—we are preparing for the specific demands of the marathon.

As marathon runners, we rely on workouts like mile repeats, two-mile repeats, or even three-mile repeats at just a hair faster than race pace to callus our legs for the marathon, the logic being that doing so will make actual race pace feel easier. And that's true to a point. I have nothing against these workouts. We do all of them at NAZ Elite, but in my view they don't simulate the feeling of those last few miles of the marathon quite like the session I am about to describe. They're more like running the first ten to twelve miles of the race, or perhaps more like miles ten to twenty, if they're done on tired legs. But what about those crucial last six miles? That's where the real problems occur for so many runners of all ages and abilities.

There is one workout that I believe can simulate those last few miles better than most. You can't do it every week, of course, nor can you do it before you're ready, before having built your fitness close to peak level with the other workouts mentioned above to create the right context for it. But if you are ready for it, there's no better way to prepare yourself for that cement-legs feeling you experience at the end of a marathon than running for two straight hours, with the first hour at a "medium" effort and the second hour at a "hard" effort. If you can deal with this feeling in the workout, and overcome it, you have a much greater chance of doing it again on race day.

On the team, we call this workout the 10/10 because, given the pace they run, the pros take about two hours to complete ten miles at medium effort followed by 10 miles at marathon effort. For the first part, I simply take their marathon pace and add fifty seconds per mile to it. That's what we run for the first half of the workout. The second half is run right at marathon pace. Because the pros all take between two to two and a half hours to complete a marathon, I use "marathon pace" and "steady state pace" interchangeably with them. For most of us, our steady state pace is faster, if not much faster, than our marathon pace.

I don't know who came up with the 10/10 originally, but I was introduced to it in reading about Terrence Mahon when he was coaching

Ryan Hall in Mammoth Lakes, California. Ryan, in the prime of his career, was one of the best runners in the world. The design of the workout made a lot of sense to me, and I certainly couldn't argue with Ryan's results. But I hesitated to try it out on my athletes because, admittedly, it seemed incredibly daunting. I was accustomed to more traditional marathon-pace sessions (which we still do), where you warm up and then run twelve to sixteen miles at marathon pace. But a few years ago I overcame my reluctance and tested the 10/10, and I'm glad I did, because I could tell right away that it had a positive effect both mentally and physically.

In 2020, we did the 10/10 exactly one month out from the Olympic Trials Marathon. Aliphine Tuliamuk, Stephanie Bruce, and Kellyn Taylor, who would go on to finish first, sixth, and eighth at the trials, all crushed it. Think about this: counting the two-mile warm-up that they started with, their twenty-second mile of the day was run at marathon effort. That right there is what makes this workout so specific.

More recently, I put the 10/10 on the schedules of several members of our team who were preparing for a marathon called the Marathon Project. As the day approached, however, we got hit by an unseasonably nasty bout of weather, with cold, rainy, windy conditions forecasted for the workout. I floated the idea of substituting the 10/10 with a different workout that would be more doable in these conditions, but the team was having none of it, so we wound up just delaying it one day and moving it to a different location, where it went off without a hitch. The fact that the runners insisted we do the 10/10 regardless of the weather says everything about how much it does for one's confidence going into a marathon.

My final note about this workout is that it is indeed very hard, as hard as I'm sure it sounds. On the occasion I just described, I gave everyone an easy four-mile run the next day to recover. So, if you choose to give it a go, remember to respect the workout and recover appropriately. If 2:09 marathoner Scott Fauble needed an easy day afterward, I think it's safe to assume you will too.

14

ULTRAMARATHON TRAINING PLANS

*I*N 2014, I SPOKE at a prerace dinner on the eve of the American River 50 Mile, a popular and highly competitive trail ultramarathon that takes place each April in Northern California. I forget why, exactly, but at one point during my talk, I asked those in the audience to raise their hand if they'd ever run the Boston Marathon. Not a single arm went up.

I was shocked. There were at least sixty runners in the room, and *none* of them had ever participated in the world's most hallowed running event? Afterward, AR50 race director Julie Fingar pulled me aside and explained to me that the whole reason ultrarunners become ultrarunners is that they're too slow to qualify for Boston. That got me thinking. At the time, I had never run an ultra, and at forty-three I was running out of new goals to chase. If what Julie said was true, I could totally kick ass at ultradistances, in which I'd had little interest previously.

I decided then and there to compete in the following year's AR50. My preparations were complicated by the fact that I lived in a flat area with poor trail access, but I figured that if I got fit enough on my usual training routes, I could dominate nevertheless.

Not so. I was served a great big slice of humble pie in my first ultramarathon, and I learned two important lessons. One was that ultras are a lot more competitive than Julie Fingar let on, and they're getting more competitive all the time. The other is that if you want to be competitive in ultramarathons, you'd better train like the most competitive ultrarunners (as I did in preparing for my second ultra, which I won). The three training plans offered in this chapter will help you do just that, whether your goal is to kick ass on the trails or you just need an alternative to the out-of-reach goal of qualifying for Boston.

Standard ultramarathon distances range from fifty kilometers to one hundred miles. The plans I've built have the flexibility to be used for any distance within this range. That's because you can't just keep training more and more to get your body ready for longer and longer events. The human body is incapable of adapting to runs exceeding roughly five hours in duration. For this reason, even elite ultrarunners specializing in the longest distances rarely do individual training runs of more than five hours, despite the fact that their races may last three or four times longer. At the other extreme, it takes at least five hours for most nonelite runners to complete a trail 50K, so they need to get close to this duration in their longest training runs. All the training plans in this chapter include a five-hour run (or run/hike for those who can't run for five hours straight), and this is why they can be used for ultramarathons of any length, though you may want to make some event-specific adjustments to whichever level you select.

The level 1 plan features four runs per week, plus two sessions that may be done either as easy runs or as nonimpact cardio cross-training sessions, and a rest day. You should be able to run comfortably for at least eighty minutes before you begin this plan. The level 2 plan features seven runs per week (six in recovery weeks), and you should be running daily for up to ninety minutes before you begin. Finally, the level 3 plan features nine runs per week (eight in recovery weeks), and you should have a solid fitness base that includes daily running and some work at higher intensities before you start it.

All three plans contain three-week step cycles, where the training load is reduced for recovery in the third week. Refer back to the Training Plans Overview for details on how to do the various workout types. Coach Ben's favorite ultramarathon workout is described in a pro tip that follows this chapter. Interactive, online versions of these training plans—plus a beginner's level 0 ultramarathon plan—are

283

available at 8020endurance.com. Adaptive versions are available through the PACE smartphone app.

• LEVEL 1 •

	MONDAY	TUESDAY	WEDNESDAY	THURSDAY	FRIDAY	SATURDAY	SUNDAY
1	Rest	Fast-Finish Run 35:00 easy 5:00 @ CV	Easy Run or Cross-Training 40:00 easy	Easy Run 40:00 easy	Fartlek Run 10:00 easy Drills and Strides 6 x 1:00 @ MAS/2:00 easy 10:00 easy	Easy Run or Cross-Training 40:00 easy	Long Run 1:20:00 easy
2	Rest	Fast-Finish Run 30:00 easy 10:00 @ LTP	Easy Run or Cross-Training 40:00 easy	Easy Run 40:00 easy	Hill-Repetitions Run 10:00 easy Drills and Strides 6 x (0:30 uphill @ VHI/1:30 easy) 10:00 easy	Easy Run or Cross-Training 40:00 easy	Long Run 1:40:00 easy
3	Rest	Fartlek Run 10:00 easy 1:00 @ 5KP 1:00 easy 2:00 @ 10KP 1:00 easy 3:00 @ HMP 1:00 easy 2:00 @ 10KP 1:00 easy 1:00 @ 5KP 10:00 easy	Easy Run or Cross-Training 40:00 easy	Easy Run 40:00 easy	Progression-Intervals Run 10:00 easy 5 x (0:30 @ SSP/0:20 @ MAS/0:10 @ VHI) 5:00 easy 5 x (0:30 @ SSP/0:20 @ MAS/0:10 @ VHI) 5:00 easy 5 x (0:30 @ SSP/0:20 @ MAS/0:10 @ VHI) 10:00 easy	Easy Run or Cross-Training 40:00 easy	Long Run 1:20:00 easy

MATT FITZGERALD AND BEN ROSARIO

	MONDAY	TUESDAY	WEDNESDAY	THURSDAY	FRIDAY	SATURDAY	SUNDAY
4	Rest	Critical-Velocity Intervals Run 10:00 easy Drills and Strides 4 x (4:00 @ CV/2:00 easy) 10:00 easy	Easy Run or Cross-Training 45:00 easy	Easy Run 45:00 easy	Hill-Repetitions Run 10:00 easy Drills and Strides 6 x (1:00 uphill @ VHI/2:00 easy) 10:00 easy	Easy Run or Cross-Training 45:00 easy	Long Run 2:00:00 easy
5	Rest	Over/Under Intervals Run 10:00 easy Drills and Strides 3 x (3:00 @ LTP plus 0:05 per mile/3:00 @ LTP-0:05 per mile/3:00 easy) 10:00 easy	Easy Run or Cross-Training 45:00 easy	Easy Run 45:00 easy	Descending-Intervals Run 10:00 easy Drills and Strides 3:00 @ MAS/2:00 easy 2:00 @ MAS/1:20 easy 1:00 @ MAS/0:40 easy 0:45 @ MAS/0:30 easy 0:30 @ MAS 10:00 easy	Easy Run or Cross-Training 45:00 easy	Long Run 1:20:00 easy
6	Rest	Progression Run 20:00 easy 12:00 @ SSP 6:00 @ LTP 3:00 @ CV 5:00 easy	Easy Run or Cross-Training 45:00 easy	Easy Run 45:00 easy	Hill-Repetitions Run 10:00 easy Drills and Strides 4 x (2:00 uphill @ HI/3:00 easy) 10:00 easy	Easy Run or Cross-Training 45:00 easy	Long Run 2:30:00 easy
7	Rest	Steady-State Run 10:00 easy Drills and Strides 30:00 @ SSP 10:00 easy	Easy Run or Cross-Training 50:00 easy	Easy Run 50:00 easy	Variable-Speed Intervals Run 10:00 easy Drills and Strides 3 x (4 x 0:30 @ MAS/0:45 @ LTP) 2:30 easy 10:00 easy	Easy Run or Cross-Training 50:00 easy	Long Run 1:40:00 easy

(Table continues)

	MONDAY	TUESDAY	WEDNESDAY	THURSDAY	FRIDAY	SATURDAY	SUNDAY
8	Rest	Relaxed 10K Time Trial 1 mile easy Drills and Strides 10K @ 10KP + 5% 1 mile easy	Easy Run or Cross-Training 50:00 easy	Easy Run 50:00 easy	Hill Repetitions Run 10:00 easy Drills and Strides 8 x (0:30 uphill @ VHI/1:30 easy) 10:00 easy	Easy Run or Cross-Training 50:00 easy	Long Run/ Hike 3:00:00 easy
9	Rest	Fartlek Run 10:00 easy 1:00 @ 5KP 1:00 easy 2:00 @ 10KP 1:00 easy 3:00 @ HMP 1:00 easy 2:00 @ 10KP 1:00 easy 1:00 @ 5KP 1:00 easy 2:00 @ 10KP 1:00 easy 3:00 @ 10KP 10:00 easy	Easy Run or Cross-Training 50:00 easy	Easy Run 50:00 easy	Progression Run 30:00 easy 8:00 @ LTP 4:00 @ CV 2:00 @ MAS 5:00 easy	Easy Run or Cross-Training 50:00 easy	Long Run 2:00:00 easy
10	Rest	Tempo Run 10:00 easy Drills and Strides 16:00 @ LTP 5:00 easy 16:00 @ LTP 10:00 easy	Easy Run or Cross-Training 55:00 easy	Easy Run 55:00 easy	Hill Repetitions Run 10:00 easy Drills and Strides 8 x (1:00 uphill @ VHI/2:00 easy) 10:00 easy	Easy Run or Cross-Training 55:00 easy	Long Run/ Hike 3:30:00 easy

MATT FITZGERALD AND BEN ROSARIO

	MONDAY	TUESDAY	WEDNESDAY	THURSDAY	FRIDAY	SATURDAY	SUNDAY
11	Rest	Steady-State Run 10:00 easy Drills and Strides 40:00 @ SSP 10:00 easy	Easy Run or Cross-Training 55:00 easy	Easy Run 55:00 easy	Accelerations Run 10:00 easy Drills and Strides 11:00 acceleration from jog to sprint 10:00 walk to jog 3:00 acceleration from jog to sprint 10:00 walk to jog	Easy Run or Cross-Training 55:00 easy	Long Run 2:00:00 easy
12	Rest	Progression Run 30:00 easy 12:00 @ SSP 6:00 @ LTP 3:00 @ CV 5:00 easy	Easy Run or Cross-Training 55:00 easy	Easy Run 55:00 easy	Hill-Repetitions Run 10:00 easy Drills and Strides 4 x (2:00 uphill @ HI/2:00 easy) 10:00 easy	Easy Run or Cross-Training 55:00 easy	Long Run/ Hike 4:00:00 easy
13	Rest	Critical- Velocity Intervals Run 10:00 easy Drills and Strides 5 x (4:00 @ CV/2:00 easy) 10:00 easy	Easy Run or Cross-Training 1:00:00 easy	Easy Run 1:00:00 easy	Lactate- Intervals Run 10:00 easy Drills and Strides 8 x (0:30 @ MAS/0:15 easy) 3:00 easy 8 x (0:30 @ MAS/0:15 easy) 3:00 easy 8 x (0:30 @ MAS/0:15 easy) 10:00 easy	Easy Run or Cross-Training 1:00:00 easy	Long Run 2:00 easy

(Table continues)

	MONDAY	TUESDAY	WEDNESDAY	THURSDAY	FRIDAY	SATURDAY	SUNDAY
14	Rest	Over/Under Intervals Run 10:00 easy Drills and Strides 3 x (4:00 @ LTP +0:05 per mile/3:00 @ LTP -0:05 per mile/2:00 easy) 10:00 easy	Easy Run or Cross-Training 1:00:00 easy	Easy Run 1:00:00 easy	Hill-Repetitions Run 10:00 easy Drills and Strides 10 x (0:30 uphill @ VHI/1:30 easy) 10:00 easy	Easy Run or Cross-Training 1:00:00 easy	Long Run/ Hike 4:30:00 easy
15	Rest	Fartlek Run 10:00 easy 1:00 @ 5KP 1:00 easy 2:00 @ 10KP 1:00 easy 3:00 @ HMP 1:00 easy 2:00 @ 10KP 1:00 easy 1:00 @ 5KP 1:00 easy 2:00 @ 10KP 1:00 easy 3:00 @ 10KP 10:00 easy	Easy Run or Cross-Training 1:00:00 easy	Easy Run 1:00:00 easy	Progression-Intervals Run 10:00 easy Drills and Strides 5 x (0:30 @ SSP/0:20 @ MAS/0:10 @ VHI) 5:00 easy 5 x (0:30 @ SSP/0:20 @ MAS/0:10 @ VHI) 5:00 easy 5 x (0:30 @ SSP/0:20 @ MAS/0:10 @ VHI) 10:00 easy	Easy Run or Cross-Training 1:00:00 easy	Long Run 2:00:00 easy
16	Rest	Steady-State Run 10:00 easy Drills and Strides 50:00 @ SSP 10:00 easy	Easy Run or Cross-Training 1:00:00 easy	Easy Run 1:00:00 easy	Hill-Repetitions Run 10:00 easy Drills and Strides 10 x (1:00 uphill @ VHI/2:00 easy) 10:00 easy	Easy Run or Cross-Training 1:00:00 easy	Long Run 5:00:00 easy

MATT FITZGERALD AND BEN ROSARIO

	MONDAY	TUESDAY	WEDNESDAY	THURSDAY	FRIDAY	SATURDAY	SUNDAY
17	Rest	Tempo Run 10:00 easy Drills and Strides 18:00 @ LTP 5:00 easy 18:00 @ LTP 10:00 easy	Easy Run or Cross-Training 1:00:00 easy	Progression Run 30:00 easy 8:00 @ LTP 4:00 @ CV 2:00 @ MAS 5:00 easy	Easy Run 1:00:00 easy	Long Run 3:00:00 easy	Long Run 2:30:00 easy
18	Rest	Fast Finish Run 50:00 easy 10:00 @ CV	Easy Run or Cross-Training 1:00:00 easy	Easy Run 1:00:00 easy	Analog- Accelerations Run 10:00 easy Drills and Strides 11:00 acceleration from jog to sprint 10:00 walk to jog 6:00 acceleration from jog to sprint 10:00 walk to jog	Easy Run 50:00 easy	Long Run 1:30:00 easy
19	Rest	Fartlek Run 10:00 easy Drills and Strides 5 x 2:00 @ in Zone 3/1:00 easy 10:00 easy	Easy Run or Cross-Training 40:00 easy	Fartlek Run 10:00 easy Drills and Strides 6 x 1:00 @ HI/2:00 easy 10:00 easy	Easy Run plus Strides 20:00 easy Drills and Strides	Ultramarathon Race	Rest

• LEVEL 2 •

	MONDAY	TUESDAY	WEDNESDAY	THURSDAY	FRIDAY	SATURDAY	SUNDAY
1	Easy Run 30:00 easy	Fast-Finish Run 45:00 easy 5:00 @ CV	Easy Run 45:00 easy	Easy Run plus Drills and Strides 45:00 easy	Fartlek Run 15:00 easy Drills and Strides 8 x 1:00 @ MAS/2:00 easy 15:00 easy	Easy Run 45:00 easy	Long Run 1:20:00 easy
2	Easy Run 30:00 easy	Fast-Finish Run 40:00 easy 10:00 @ LTP	Easy Run 45:00 easy	Easy Run plus Drills and Strides 45:00 easy	Hill-Repetitions Run 15:00 easy Drills and Strides 8 x (0:30 uphill @ VHI/1:30 easy) 15:00 easy	Easy Run 45:00 easy	Long Run 1:40:00 easy
3	Rest	Fartlek Run 15:00 easy 1:00 @ 5KP 1:00 easy 2:00 @ 10KP 1:00 easy 3:00 @ HMP 1:00 easy 2:00 @ 10KP 1:00 easy 1:00 @ 5KP 1:00 easy 2:00 @ 10KP 1:00 easy 3:00 @ HMP 15:00 easy	Easy Run 45:00 easy	Easy Run plus Drills and Strides 45:00 easy	Progression-Intervals Run 15:00 easy Drills and Strides 5 x (0:30 @ SSP/0:20 @ MAS/0:10 @ VHI) 5:00 easy 5 x (0:30 @ SSP/0:20 @ MAS/0:10 @ VHI) 5:00 easy 5 x (0:30 @ SSP/0:20 @ MAS/0:10 @ VHI) 15:00 easy	Easy Run 45:00 easy	Long Run 1:20:00 easy

	MONDAY	TUESDAY	WEDNESDAY	THURSDAY	FRIDAY	SATURDAY	SUNDAY
4	Easy Run 30:00 easy	Critical-Velocity Intervals Run 15:00 easy Drills and Strides 5 x (4:00 @ CV/2:00 easy) 15:00 easy	Easy Run 50:00 easy	Easy Run plus Drills and Strides 50:00 easy Drills and Strides	Hill Repetitions Run 15:00 easy Drills and Strides 5 x (2:00 uphill @ HI/3:00 easy) 15:00 easy	Easy Run 50:00 easy	Long Run 2:00:00 easy
5	Easy Run 30:00 easy	Over/Under Intervals Run 15:00 easy Drills and Strides 3 x (4:00 @ LTP plus 0:05 per mile/3:00 @ LTP-0:05 per mile/2:00 easy) 15:00 easy	Easy Run 50:00 easy	Easy Run plus Drills and Strides 50:00 easy Drills and Strides	Descending-Intervals Run 15:00 easy Drills and Strides 3:00 @ MAS/2:00 easy 2:00 @ MAS/1:20 easy 1:00 @ MAS/0:40 easy 0:45 @ MAS/0:30 easy 0:30 @ MAS 0:45 @ MAS/0:30 easy 0:30 @ MAS 15:00 easy	Easy Run 50:00 easy	Long Run 2:15:00 easy
6	Rest	Progression Run 20:00 easy 16:00 @ SSP 8:00 @ LTP 4:00 @ CV 5:00 easy	Easy Run 50:00 easy	Easy Run plus Drills and Strides 50:00 easy Drills and Strides	Hill-Repetitions Run 15:00 easy Drills and Strides 8 x (1:00 uphill @ VHI/2:00 easy) 15:00 easy	Easy Run 50:00 easy	Long Run 1:30:00 easy

(Table continues)

	MONDAY	TUESDAY	WEDNESDAY	THURSDAY	FRIDAY	SATURDAY	SUNDAY
7	Easy Run 30:00 easy	Steady-State Run 15:00 easy Drills and Strides 40:00 @ SSP 15:00 easy	Easy Run 55:00 easy	Easy Run plus Drills and Strides 55:00 easy Drills and Strides	Variable-Speed Intervals Run 15:00 easy Drills and Strides 4 x (4 x 0:30 @ MAS/0:45 @ LTP) 2:30 easy 15:00 easy	Easy Run 55:00 easy	Long Run 2:30:00 easy
8	Easy Run 30:00 easy	Relaxed 10K Time Trial 1.5 miles easy Drills and strides 10K @ 10KP + 5% 1.5 miles easy	Easy Run 55:00 easy	Easy Run plus Drills and Strides 55:00 easy Drills and Strides	Hill-Repetitions Run 15:00 easy Drills and Strides 10 x (0:30 uphill @ VHI/1:30 easy) 15:00 easy	Easy Run 55:00 easy	Long Run 3:00:00 easy
9	Rest	Fartlek Run 15:00 easy 1:00 @ 5KP 1:00 easy 2:00 @ 10KP 1:00 easy 3:00 @ HMP 1:00 easy 2:00 @ 10KP 1:00 easy 1:00 @ 5KP 1:00 easy 2:00 @ 10KP 1:00 easy 3:00 @ HMP 15:00 easy	Easy Run 55:00 easy	Easy Run plus Drills and Strides 55:00 easy Drills and Strides	Progression Run 20:00 easy 12:00 @ LTP 6:00 @ CV 3:00 @ MAS 5:00 easy	Easy Run 55:00 easy	Long Run 1:45:00 easy
10	Easy Run 30:00 easy	Tempo Run 15:00 easy Drills and Strides 18:00 @ LTP 5:00 easy 18:00 @ LTP 15:00 easy	Easy Run 1:00:00 easy	Easy Run plus Drills and Strides 1:00:00 easy Drills and Strides	Hill-Repetitions Run 15:00 easy Drills and Strides 6 x (2:00 uphill @ HI/3:00 easy) 15:00 easy	Easy Run 1:00:00 easy	Long Run 3:30:00 easy

	MONDAY	TUESDAY	WEDNESDAY	THURSDAY	FRIDAY	SATURDAY	SUNDAY
11	Easy Run 30:00 easy	Steady-State Run 15:00 easy Drills and Strides 50:00 @ SSP 15:00 easy	Easy Run 1:00:00 easy	Analog-Accelerations Run 15:00 easy Drills and Strides 11:00 acceleration from jog to sprint 10:00 walk to jog 6:00 acceleration from jog to sprint 15:00 walk to jog	Easy Run plus Drills and Strides 1:00:00 easy Drills and Strides	Long Run 1:45:00 easy	Long Run 1:45:00 easy
12	Rest	Progression Run 30:00 easy 16:00 @ SSP 8:00 @ LTP 4:00 @ CV 5:00 easy	Easy Run 1:00:00 easy	Easy Run plus Drills and Strides 1:00:00 easy Drills and Strides	Hill-Repetitions Run 15:00 easy Drills and Strides 6 x (2:00 uphill @ HI/3:00 easy) 15:00 easy	Easy Run 1:00:00 easy	Long Run 2:00:00 easy
13	Easy Run 30:00 easy	Critical-Velocity Intervals Run 15:00 easy Drills and Strides 6 x (4:00 @ CV/2:00 easy) 15:00 easy	Easy Run 1:00:00 easy	Easy Run plus Drills and Strides 1:05:00 easy Drills and Strides	Lactate-Intervals run 15:00 easy Drills and Strides 10 x (0:30 @ MAS/0:15 easy) 3:00 easy 10 x (0:30 @ MAS/0:15 easy) 3:00 easy 10 x (0:30 @ MAS/0:15 easy) 15:00 easy	Easy Run 1:00:00 easy	Long Run 4:30:00 easy

(Table continues)

	MONDAY	TUESDAY	WEDNESDAY	THURSDAY	FRIDAY	SATURDAY	SUNDAY
14	Easy Run 30:00 easy	Over/Under Intervals Run 15:00 easy Drills and Strides 4 x (3:00 @ LTP plus 0:05 per mile/3:00 @ LTP-0:05 per mile/3:00 easy) 15:00 easy	Easy Run 1:00:00 easy	Hill-Repetitions Run 15:00 easy Drills and Strides 8 x (1:00 uphill @ VHI/2:00 easy) 15:00 easy	Easy Run plus Drills and Strides 1:05:00 easy Drills and Strides	Long Run 2:00:00 easy	Long Run 2:00:00 easy
15	Rest	Progression Run 40:00 easy 12:00 @ SSP 8:00 @ LTP 4:00 @ CV 5:00 easy	Easy Run 1:00:00 easy	Easy Run plus Drills and Strides 1:05:00 easy Drills and Strides	Progression-Intervals Run 15:00 easy Drills and Strides 5 x (0:30 @ SSP/0:20 @ MAS/0:10 @ VHI) 5:00 easy 5 x (0:30 @ SSP/0:20 @ MAS/0:10 @ VHI) 5:00 easy 5 x (0:30 @ SSP/0:20 @ MAS/0:10 @ VHI) 15:00 easy	Easy Run 1:00:00 easy	Long Run 2:00:00 easy
16	Easy Run 30:00 easy	Steady-State Run 15:00 easy Drills and Strides 1:00:00 @ SSP 15:00 easy	Easy Run 1:00:00 easy	Easy Run plus Drills and Strides 1:10:00 easy Drills and Strides	Hill-Repetitions Run 15:00 easy Drills and Strides 6 x (2:00 uphill @ HI/3:00 easy) 15:00 easy	Easy Run 1:00:00 easy	Long Run 5:00:00 easy

294

	MONDAY	TUESDAY	WEDNESDAY	THURSDAY	FRIDAY	SATURDAY	SUNDAY
17	Easy Run 30:00 easy	Tempo Run 15:00 easy Drills and Strides 22:00 @ LTP 5:00 easy 22:00 @ LTP 15:00 easy	Easy Run 1:00:00 easy	Progression Run 20:00 easy 12:00 @ LTP 6:00 @ CV 3:00 @ MAS 5:00 easy	Easy Run 1:00:00 easy	Long Run 3:15:00 easy	Long Run 2:45:00 easy
18	Rest	Fast-Finish Run 1:00:00 easy 10:00 @ CV	Easy Run 1:00:00 easy	Easy Run plus Drills and Strides 1:00:00 easy Drills and Strides	Analog-Accelerations Run 15:00 easy Drills and Strides 11:00 acceleration from jog to sprint 10:00 walk to jog 6:00 acceleration from jog to sprint 15:00 walk to jog	Easy Run 55:00 easy	Long Run 1:45:00 easy
19	Easy Run 30:00 easy	Fartlek Run 15:00 easy Drills and Strides 6 x 2:00 @ in Zone 3/1:00 easy 15:00 easy	Easy Run 45:00 easy	Easy Run 40:00 easy	Fartlek Run 10:00 easy Drills and Strides 8 x 1:00 @ HI/2:00 easy 10:00 easy	Easy Run plus Strides 20:00 easy Drills and Strides	Ultramarathon Race

· LEVEL 3 ·

	MONDAY	TUESDAY	WEDNESDAY	THURSDAY	FRIDAY	SATURDAY	SUNDAY
1	Easy Run 40:00 easy	Fast-Finish Run 55:00 easy 5:00 @ CV	Easy Run 1:00:00 easy	Easy Run plus Drills, Strides, and Plyos 1:00:00 easy Drills, Strides, and Plyos	Fartlek Run 20:00 easy Drills and Strides 10 x 1:00 @ MAS/2:00 easy 20:00 easy	Easy Run 1:00:00 easy	Long Run 1:40:00 easy
		Easy Run 20:00 easy			Easy Run 20:00 easy		
2	Easy Run 40:00 easy	Fast-Finish Run 50:00 easy 10:00 @ LTP	Easy Run 1:00:00 easy	Easy Run plus Drills, Strides, and Plyos 1:00:00 easy Drills, Strides, and Plyos	Hill-Repetitions Run 20:00 easy Drills and Strides 10 x (0:30 uphill @ VHI/1:30 easy) 20:00 easy	Easy Run 1:00:00 easy	Long Run 2:00:00 easy
		Easy Run 25:00 easy			Easy Run 25:00 easy		
3	Rest	Fartlek Run 20:00 easy 1:00 @ 5KP 1:00 easy 2:00 @ 10KP 1:00 easy 3:00 @ HMP 1:00 easy 2:00 @ 10KP 1:00 easy 1:00 @ 5KP 1:00 easy 2:00 @ 10KP 1:00 easy 3:00 @ HMP 20:00 easy	Easy Run 1:00:00 easy	Easy Run plus Drills, Strides, and Plyos 1:00:00 easy Drills, Strides, and Plyos	Progression Intervals Run 20:00 easy Drills and Strides 5 x (0:30 @ SSP/0:20 @ MAS/0:10 @ VHI) 5:00 easy 5 x (0:30 @ SSP/0:20 @ MAS/0:10 @ VHI) 5:00 easy 5 x (0:30 @ SSP/0:20 @ MAS/0:10 @ VHI) 20:00 easy	Easy Run 1:00:00 easy	Long Run 1:30:00 easy
		Easy Run 20:00 easy			Easy Run 20:00 easy		

MATT FITZGERALD AND BEN ROSARIO

	MONDAY	TUESDAY	WEDNESDAY	THURSDAY	FRIDAY	SATURDAY	SUNDAY
4	Easy Run 40:00 easy	Critical-Velocity Intervals Run 20:00 easy Drills and Strides 6 x 4:00 @ CV/2:00 easy 20:00 easy Easy Run 25:00 easy	Easy Run 1:00:00 easy	Easy Run plus Drills, Strides, and Plyos 1:05:00 easy Drills, Strides, and Plyos	Hill-Repetitions Run 20:00 easy Drills and Strides 6 x (2:00 uphill @ HI/2:00 easy) 20:00 easy Easy Run 25:00 easy	Easy Run 1:00:00 easy	Long Run 2:15:00 easy
5	Easy Run 40:00 easy	Over/Under Intervals Run 20:00 easy Drills and Strides 4 x (3:00 @ LTP plus 0:05 per mile/3:00 @ LTP-0:05 per mile/3:00 easy) 20:00 easy Easy Run 30:00 easy	Easy Run 1:00:00 easy	Easy Run plus Drills, Strides, and Plyos 1:05:00 easy Drills, Strides, and Plyos	Descending-Intervals Run 20:00 easy Drills and Strides 3:00 @ MAS/2:00 easy 2:00 @ MAS/1:20 easy 1:00 @ MAS/0:40 easy 0:45 @ MAS/0:30 easy 0:30 @ MAS 0:45 @ MAS/0:30 easy 0:30 @ MAS 20:00 easy Easy Run 30:00 easy	Easy Run 1:00:00 easy	Long Run 2:30:00 easy

(Table continues)

RUN LIKE A PRO (EVEN IF YOU'RE SLOW)

	MONDAY	TUESDAY	WEDNESDAY	THURSDAY	FRIDAY	SATURDAY	SUNDAY
6	Rest	Progression Run 30:00 easy 16:00 @ SSP 8:00 @ LTP 4:00 @ CV 5:00 easy Easy Run 25:00 easy	Easy Run 1:00:00 easy	Easy Run plus Drills, Strides, and Plyos 1:05:00 easy Drills, Strides, and Plyos	Hill Repetitions Run 20:00 easy Drills and Strides 10 x (1:00 uphill @ VHI/2:00 easy) 20:00 easy Easy Run 25:00 easy	Easy Run 1:00:00 easy	Long Run 2:00:00 easy
7	Easy Run 40:00 easy	Steady-State Run 20:00 easy Drills and Strides 45:00 @ SSP 20:00 easy Easy Run 30:00 easy	Easy Run 1:00:00 easy	Easy Run plus Drills, Strides, and Plyos 1:10:00 easy Drills, Strides, and Plyos	Variable-Speed Intervals Run 20:00 easy Drills and Strides 5 x (4 x 0:30 @ MAS/0:45 @ LTP) 2:30 easy 20:00 easy Easy Run 30:00 easy	Easy Run 1:00:00 easy	Long Run 2:45:00 easy
8	Easy Run 40:00 easy	Relaxed 10K Time Trial 2 miles easy Drills and strides 10K @ 10KP plus 5 percent 2 miles easy Easy Run 35:00 easy	Easy Run 1:00:00 easy	Easy Run plus Drills, Strides, and Plyos 1:10:00 easy Drills, Strides, and Plyos	Hill Repetitions Run 20:00 easy Drills and Strides 12 x (0:30 uphill @ VHI/1:30 easy) 20:00 easy Easy Run 35:00 easy	Easy Run 1:00:00 easy	Long Run 3:00:00 easy

	MONDAY	TUESDAY	WEDNESDAY	THURSDAY	FRIDAY	SATURDAY	SUNDAY
9	Rest	Fartlek Run 20:00 easy 1:00 @ 5KP 1:00 easy 2:00 @ 10KP 1:00 easy 3:00 @ HMP 1:00 easy 2:00 @ 10KP 1:00 easy 1:00 @ 5KP 1:00 easy 2:00 @ 10KP 1:00 easy 3:00 @ HMP 1:00 easy 2:00 @ 10KP 1:00 easy 1:00 @ 5KP 20:00 easy Easy Run 30:00 easy	Easy Run 1:00:00 easy	Easy Run plus Drills, Strides, and Plyos 1:10:00 easy Drills, Strides, and Plyos	Progression Run 30:00 easy 12:00 @ LTP 6:00 @ CV 3:00 @ MAS 5:00 easy Easy Run 30:00 easy	Easy Run 1:00:00 easy	Depletion Run 2:00:00 easy, no calories before or during
10	Easy Run 40:00 easy	Tempo Run 20:00 easy Drills and Strides 20:00 @ LTP 5:00 easy 20:00 @ LTP 20:00 easy Easy Run 35:00 easy	Easy Run 1:00:00 easy	Easy Run plus Drills, Strides, and Plyos 1:15:00 easy Drills, Strides, and Plyos	Hill Repetitions Run 20:00 easy Drills and Strides 7 x (2:00 uphill @ HI/2:00 easy) 20:00 easy Easy Run 35:00 easy	Easy Run 1:00:00 easy	Long Run 3:30:00 easy

(Table continues)

	MONDAY	TUESDAY	WEDNESDAY	THURSDAY	FRIDAY	SATURDAY	SUNDAY
11	Easy Run 40:00 easy	Steady-State Run 20:00 easy Drills and Strides 55:00 @ SSP 20:00 easy Easy Run 35:00 easy	Easy Run 1:00:00 easy	Accelerations Run 20:00 easy Drills and Strides 11:00 acceleration from jog to sprint 10:00 walk to jog 6:00 acceleration from jog to sprint 10:00 walk to jog 3:00 acceleration from jog to sprint 20:00 walk to jog Easy Run 35:00 easy	Easy Run plus Drills, Strides, and Plyos 1:15:00 easy Drills, Strides, and Plyos	Long Run 2:00:00 easy	Long Run 2:00:00 easy
12	Rest	Progression Run 35:00 easy 16:00 @ SSP 8:00 @ LTP 4:00 @ CV 5:00 easy Easy Run 30:00 easy	Easy Run 1:00:00 easy	Easy Run plus Drills, Strides, and Plyos 1:15:00 easy Drills, Strides, and Plyos	Hill-Repetitions Run 20:00 easy Drills and Strides 10 x (1:00 uphill @ VHI/2:00 easy) 20:00 easy Easy Run 30:00 easy	Easy Run 1:00:00 easy	Depletion Run 2:20:00 easy, no calories before or during

	MONDAY	TUESDAY	WEDNESDAY	THURSDAY	FRIDAY	SATURDAY	SUNDAY
13	Easy Run 40:00 easy	Critical Velocity Intervals Run 20:00 easy Drills and Strides 7 x (4:00 @ CV/2:00 easy) 20:00 easy Easy Run 35:00 easy	Easy Run 1:00:00 easy	Easy Run plus Drills, Strides, and Plyos 1:15:00 easy Drills, Strides, and Plyos	Lactate Intervals run 20:00 easy Drills and Strides 12 x (0:30 @ MAS/0:15 easy) 3:00 easy 12 x (0:30 @ MAS/0:15 easy) 3:00 easy 12 x (0:30 @ MAS/0:15 easy) 20:00 easy Easy Run 35:00 easy	Easy Run 1:00:00 easy	Long Run 4:30:00 easy
14	Easy Run 40:00 easy	Over/Under Intervals Run 20:00 easy Drills and Strides 4 x (4:00 @ LTP plus 0:05 per mile/3:00 @ LTP-0:05 per mile/2:00 easy) 20:00 easy Easy Run 35:00 easy	Easy Run 1:00:00 easy	Hill-Repetitions Run 20:00 easy Drills and Strides 12 x (0:30 uphill @ VHI/1:30 easy) 20:00 easy Easy Run 35:00 easy	Easy Run plus Drills, Strides, and Plyos 1:15:00 easy Drills, Strides, and Plyos	Depletion Run 2:30:00 easy, no calories before or during	Long Run 2:30:00 easy

(Table continues)

	MONDAY	TUESDAY	WEDNESDAY	THURSDAY	FRIDAY	SATURDAY	SUNDAY
15	Rest	Fartlek Run 20:00 easy 1:00 @ 5KP 1:00 easy 2:00 @ 10KP 1:00 easy 3:00 @ HMP 1:00 easy 2:00 @ 10KP 1:00 easy 1:00 @ 5KP 1:00 easy 2:00 @ 10KP 1:00 easy 3:00 @ HMP 1:00 easy 2:00 @ 10KP 1:00 easy 1:00 @ 5KP 20:00 easy Easy Run 30:00 easy	Easy Run 1:00:00 easy	Easy Run plus Drills, Strides, and Plyos 1:15:00 easy Drills, Strides, and Plyos	Progression Intervals Run 20:00 easy Drills and Strides 5 x (0:30 @ SSP/0:20 @ MAS/0:10 @ VHI) 5:00 easy 5 x (0:30 @ SSP/0:20 @ MAS/0:10 @ VHI) 5:00 easy 5 x (0:30 @ SSP/0:20 @ MAS/0:10 @ VHI) 5:00 easy 5 x (0:30 @ SSP/0:20 @ MAS/0:10 @ VHI) 20:00 easy Easy Run 30:00 easy	Easy Run 1:00:00 easy	Depletion Run 2:40:00 easy, no calories before or during
16	Easy Run 40:00 easy	Steady-State Run 20:00 easy Drills and Strides 1:05:00 @ SSP 20:00 easy Easy Run 35:00 easy	Easy Run 1:00:00 easy	Easy Run plus Drills, Strides, and Plyos 1:15:00 easy Drills, Strides, and Plyos	Hill- Repetitions Run 20:00 easy Drills and Strides 7 x (2:00 uphill @ HI/2:00 easy) 20:00 easy Easy Run 35:00 easy	Easy Run 1:00:00 easy	Long Run 5:00:00 easy

	MONDAY	TUESDAY	WEDNESDAY	THURSDAY	FRIDAY	SATURDAY	SUNDAY
17	Easy Run 40:00 easy	Tempo Run 20:00 easy Drills and Strides 24:00 @ LTP 5:00 easy 24:00 @ LTP 20:00 easy Easy Run 35:00 easy	Easy Run 1:00:00 easy	Descending Intervals Run 20:00 easy Drills and Strides 3:00 @ MAS/2:00 easy 2:00 @ MAS/1:20 easy 1:00 @ MAS/0:40 easy 0:45 @ MAS/0:30 easy 0:30 @ MAS 0:45 @ MAS/0:30 easy 0:30 @ MAS 20:00 easy Easy Run 35:00 easy	Easy Run plus Drills, Strides, and Plyos 1:15:00 easy Drills, Strides, and Plyos	Coach Ben's Favorite Ultramarathon Workout 3:30:00 easy, no calories before or during	Coach Ben's Favorite Ultramarathon Workout 3:00:00 easy
18	Rest	Critical-Velocity Intervals Run 20:00 easy Drills and Strides 6 x (4:00 @ CV/2:00 easy) 20:00 easy Easy Run 30:00 easy	Easy Run 1:00:00 easy	Easy Run plus Drills, Strides, and Plyos 1:00:00 easy Drills, Strides, and Plyos	Progression Run 30:00 easy 12:00 @ LTP 6:00 @ CV 3:00 @ MAS 5:00 easy Easy Run 30:00 easy	Easy Run 1:00:00 easy	Long Run 2:00:00 easy
19	Easy Run 40:00 easy	Fartlek Run 20:00 easy Drills and Strides 7 x 2:00 @ LTP/1:00 easy 20:00 easy	Easy Run 1:00:00 easy	Fartlek Run 20:00 easy Drills and Strides 10 x 1:00 @ MAS/2:00 easy 20:00 easy	Easy Run 40:00 easy	Easy Run plus Strides 20:00 easy Drills and Strides	Ultramarathon Race

303

My Favorite Ultramarathon Workout

Back-to-Back Long Runs; three to four hours on day one and two to three hours on day two.

Confession: When I moved to Flagstaff in 2012, I knew nothing about the world of ultramarathoning. I had never heard of Western States, or Leadville, or UTMB, and the only Hard Rock I knew of was a hotel—not a one-hundred-miler. I was clueless. Fast-forward a few years, and now I coach a team that is sponsored by one of the most prominent shoe brands in all of ultrarunning, I've been on runs with Jim Walmsley, I've watched Western States in person (and loved it), and I can now explain, in detail, the meaning of Rim-to-Rim-to-Rim.

By the way, if you are as clueless as I was, Western States, Leadville, and Hard Rock are America's most famous one-hundred-mile races, UTMB is a week-long ultramarathon extravaganza in France, and Jim Walmsley is arguably the best ultrarunner in US history. Oh yeah, and Rim-to-Rim-to-Rim is a well-known challenge in the ultramarathoning world where runners take off from the South Rim of the Grand Canyon and run to the North Rim and back (forty-two miles). Walmsley has the fastest known time (FKT) of five hours, fifty-five minutes, twenty seconds.

I've also gotten to know a few of the top young ultra stars, including Stephen Kersh, who finished seventh at Western States in 2019 and was the runner-up at the JFK fifty-miler in 2020. I went to Kersh for advice on what to write about in this tip. I told him I wanted something basic and fundamental—something that, like the workouts I shared in the previous few tips, was practical and effective.

The answer came quickly: back-to-back long runs. Rarely practiced by track and road racers, back-to-back long runs are a key weapon in the arsenal of nearly all of the top ultrarunners. They make a heck of a lot of sense, because if you're trying to prepare the body for the rigors of running fifty kilometers, or one hundred kilometers, or one hundred miles, you need to get used to being on your feet for a long time. However, because there are only so many hours in the day, and because the body can only handle so much, it isn't practical to go out for long runs of fifty miles or more—at least not very often. So you have to do the next best thing and cover a lot of ground, but do it over the course of a weekend instead of a single day.

An ideal weekend of back-to-back long runs might look something like this: first, you study the terrain you are going to be facing in your goal ultramarathon. Let's say, for example, it's going to be super hilly with lots of single-track trails. Ultrarunning race directors always seem to be seeking out the hardest routes possible, so this description is a pretty safe bet. Then, you search for similar terrain in your neck of the woods. We can't all live in Flagstaff, so this may take some work, but where there's a will, there's a way. Next, you plan out routes for both Saturday and Sunday that, combined, will take you five to seven hours to complete. Finally, you prepare for those runs diligently because this isn't your weekend long run around your local park. You'll need a fueling plan, a safety plan, a recovery plan, and preferably a partner as well.

In addition to the planning, the actual execution of the runs is quite different than you may be used to. Gone are the mile markers and splits. Now it's all about vert (a.k.a. total vertical gain over the course of the run). Gone also is the expectation of a run that starts off slowly, gradually gets faster, and inevitably finishes with an overall negative split. Instead, depending on the terrain, you may have giant fluctuations in pace throughout the run. In fact, parts of the run may not involve running. Steep inclines may force you into a fast walk, or a hike. These things are all a part of ultrarunning.

And while athletes like Kersh and Walmsley may be pushing the boundaries of speed in the ultraworld, most nonelite ultrarunners should be focused first and foremost on callusing the body for the rigors of a race that is going to take ten, fifteen, even twenty-four hours or more. That's why the second day of the back-to-back long run is so important. You are beginning that run with a deficit. After what was no doubt an exhausting Saturday, you have to wake up on Sunday and do it all over again. This is why Sunday mimics the race itself way more than Saturday. You'll be fighting physical issues— things like blisters, cramps, and various aches and pains—but perhaps most of all, you'll be fighting the signals in your mind telling you the body has had enough, that it's time to quit, that you should call it early. Overriding these signals (unless they are true emergencies) will be essential practice for race day. Sure, it's a grind, but that's what you signed up for—so embrace it!

ABOUT THE AUTHORS

MATT FITZGERALD is an acclaimed endurance sportswriter, coach, and certified sports nutritionist. He has authored or coauthored more than twenty-five books, including *The Comeback Quotient*, *Running the Dream*, and *How Bad Do You Want It?* Also an award-winning journalist, he has written for *Bicycling*, *Maxim*, *Men's Journal*, *Outside Magazine*, *Runner's World*, *Shape Magazine*, *Triathlete*, and other major magazines and websites.

An All-State runner in high school and an All-American triathlete as an adult, he continues to compete at a high level as both a runner and a triathlete. He has coached other endurance athletes since 2001. He is a cofounder of 80/20 Endurance, an Internet-based training resource for runners and other athletes.

BEN ROSARIO is the head coach of the HOKA NAZ Elite professional distance running team in Flagstaff, Arizona. His athletes have finished in the top ten of the Boston, Chicago, New York City, and London marathons, and they have won multiple national titles including the 2020 Olympic Trials Marathon. Before founding NAZ Elite, he co-owned Big River Running Company, a run-specialty store in his hometown of Saint Louis, Missouri. Ben has coauthored two previous running books, *Inside A Marathon* and *Tradition, Class, Pride*.

Ready to find
your next great read?

Let us help.

Visit prh.com/nextread

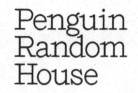